KETO DIET

FOR

WOMEN

OVER 50

The complete ketogenic dietary guide

for beginners, burn fat, weight loss,

diabetes prevention, hormonal support

Felicity Healthy

CONTENTS

Recording of this publication is strictly prohibited and any storage of this document is not allowed unless with written permission from the publisher. All rights reserved.

The information provided herein is stated to be truthful and consistent, in that any liability, in terms of inattention or otherwise, by any usage or abuse of any policies, processes, or directions contained within is the solitary and utter responsibility of the recipient reader. Under no circumstances will any legal responsibility or blame be held against the publisher for any reparation, damages, or monetary loss due to the information herein, either directly or indirectly.

Respective authors own all copyrights not held by the publisher.

The information herein is offered for informational purposes solely and is universal as so. The presentation of the information is without a contract or any type of guarantee assurance. The trademarks that are used are without any consent, and the publication of the trademark is without permission or backing by the trademark owner. All trademarks and brands within this book are for clarifying purposes only and are owned by the owners themselves, not affiliated with this document.

PROBLEMS IN WOMEN OVER THE AGE OF 50 YEARS OLD

The female body is one of the most complex systems in nature, which over the years begins to malfunction. These complex - age-related changes in the body manifest themselves in the form of hormonal changes and further exacerbation of existing chronic diseases. What gynecological problems can a woman over 60 faces?

In fact, a woman's health after 50 years is largely curled by herself. In order to feel energy, vitality and a surge of vitality, it is necessary to adhere to proper nutrition from youth, lead an active lifestyle, enjoy every new day and, of course, do not forget about regular visits to the antenatal clinic. After all, only with constant preventive examinations can you detect or prevent any serious disease in time. What gynecological diseases can occur in women after 50 years? Each of us must know this.

Involuntary urination. This phenomenon is often found in women after 60 years, and this is due to a weakening of the muscles of the sphincter of the bladder. Not an exception is the problem of prolapse of the internal female organs - the uterus, rectum, and vagina, which, however, can be found. In order to avoid trouble, it is necessary to train the muscles of the pelvic floor from a young age, namely, to perform certain exercises daily to strengthen internal organs.

Cyst. Menopause ovarian cysts are not so rare. The cause of this pathology can be many things, ranging from the age category to inflammatory processes, infertility, as well as malfunctions in the functioning of the ovaries and uterine diseases. Some cysts need to be simply observed, and some neoplasms should be urgently removed, but the attending physician decides all this.

Inflammatory processes. Female inflammatory diseases after 60 years include vaginitis, vulvovaginitis, endometritis, and so on. They can appear both against the background of infectious and viral foci (chlamydia, gonorrhea, trichomoniasis), and may form from the outside, against the background of imbalance in hormonal activity. At the same time, a woman can feel quite healthy, and vice versa. A doctor who has previously established the type of pathogen and has prescribed the necessary treatment will help to solve this problem.

Oncology. The tendency to cancer increases more in women who are over 60, but not an exception, and other ages. There is a cancer of the cervix uterus, cancer of the uterus, ovaries, and vagina, which in the early stages cannot be determined without examination. Malignant tumors make themselves felt - they are accompanied by pains in the lower abdomen, bloody discharge. Genital cancer along with breast cancer takes the second - third place in the structure of causes of mortality in women.

Menopause

I saved this for last in this section because it is the most common and inevitable fate of all women.

Aging is a genetically programmed process. Meanwhile, over the last half-century, the life expectancy of a woman has changed significantly after the onset of menopause. By the end of the 20th century, women spend almost a third of their lives in a postmenopausal state, which determines the importance of the medical and social problems of this age group of the population for society. The projected life expectancy of women 10 years ago is 80 years or more.

Causes of Menopause

Menopause occurs at the moment when the ovaries cease to function in the female body and there is a significant decrease in the levels of two hormones produced by the ovaries (estrogen and progesterone). This is a gradual process that lasts for several years and is called "perimenopause". During perimenopause, menstruation often becomes irregular, and the cycle duration changes. At the heart of this is a sharp decrease in the synthesis of hormones in the ovaries. Sex hormones are known to exert effects on various organs and tissues through binding to specific receptors. These receptors are localized in the uterus, mammary glands, in the cells of the genitourinary tract, bone tissue, brain, heart, and arteries, in the skin and its appendages, mucous membranes. Against the background of a lack of sex hormones, the so-called climacteric disorders occur, characterized by the appearance of "hot flashes", sweating, heart attacks, headaches, increased irritability, sleep disturbance and working capacity, depression. The woman notes with anxiety the loss of skin elasticity, the rapid appearance of wrinkles, dryness, and pain during sexual activity. Dysuric disorders (frequent urination), pain in bones, joints, muscles, physical activity decreases, and age-related obesity progresses. The appearance of unpleasant symptoms and especially the occurrence of irregular bleeding from the genital tract means that a woman needs to consult a doctor and discuss the occurrence of a problem. Although some women undergo menopause without any troubles, it's known

Clinical manifestations

Symptoms can be divided into distant and closest, associated with effects on blood vessels, bones, skin, and genitals.

Immediate symptoms

Vascular (hot flashes and night sweats) are the most common menopausal symptoms. During perimenopause, three out of four women experience a sudden unpleasant sensation of heat spreading across the face, neck, and chest, and in rare cases throughout the body. This sensation may be accompanied by sweating and chills. Attacks can occur at any time of the day or night from one to one hundred times a week and last from several minutes to half an hour. Most of these attacks last about three minutes. These symptoms can last for several years and are so pronounced that they begin to interfere with normal sleep and everyday life. Some women also describe unpleasant tingling sensations throughout the body. Both hot flashes and other symptoms can disappear when prescribing a special treatment - hormone replacement therapy (HRT).

Musculoskeletal

Leather. Due to the fact that the skin loses protein, called collagen, it becomes thinner, dry, wrinkled. Loss of shape and resilience also appears in other estrogen-dependent organs, such as mammary glands. The skin is more prone to bruising and scratching. Axillary and pubic hair can become thinner, and on the face in some cases, on the contrary, hair growth is enhanced. HRT helps maintain collagen levels and therefore slows down these processes.

Joint and bone pain. Some perimenopausal women complain of acute pain and aching joints. This may be due to the increase in bone fragility characteristics of this period. (We'll talk about this in more detail in the section on osteoporosis.)

Genitourinary

In the postmenopausal period, the vaginal mucosa, like the mammary glands, becomes thinner and drier, which leads to soreness during intercourse, which in turn can affect their frequency. These symptoms can be reduced by local means, which gives a short-term effect, so it is better to carry out HRT, which affects the cause of these phenomena. Since urinary tract tissue also thins, postmenopausal women are often worried about functional disorders of the bladder, such as sudden urination or coughing, sneezing, or stress (stress urinary incontinence). These symptoms can also be corrected by HRT.

Psychological

Many problems in the emotional sphere that arise in middle age (the "midlife crisis") are mistakenly associated with menopause. At this time, domestic and emotional problems in the family may appear, such as growing up children, problems associated with work or poor health. It is often possible to get rid of the problems of the "midlife crisis" after consulting a psychologist. A good doctor and support from her husband and family are more beneficial for a woman than sedatives. There is no doubt, however, that menopause can lead to mood swings, forgetfulness, loss of attention, insomnia, and depression, all of these symptoms diminishing after the appointment of HRT.

Decreased libido. Studies show that in at least a third of postmenopausal women, interest in sex is dying out. In most cases, this is caused by changes in the body associated with menopause (dryness of the vaginal mucosa, etc.), and in some cases, a decreased level of hormones affects the sex life. Using HRT will help solve these problems.

During perimenopause, women can still become pregnant if they do not use contraceptives. However, as soon as menstruation has completely stopped, pregnancy can no longer occur, because of the ovaries no longer function, even if some types of HRT cause regular monthly bleeding.

Distant symptoms

Osteoporosis. Probably the most serious long-term consequence of menopause is osteoporosis or bone fragility. Bones reach their maximum density by age 40, after which gradual bone loss begins. This process proceeds faster in women than in men, and loss occurs at a rate of 2-3% of bone mass per year since the onset of menopause. As a result, the incidence of bone fractures, especially bones of the spine (vertebrae), wrists and femoral neck, increases. If untreated, almost 50% of women undergo fractures in one place or another by the age of 70. Fractures of the vertebrae lead to unbearable pain, disability, a significant decrease in their own growth and deformation of the spine, known as the "widow's hump". Fractures of the femoral neck in women in the postmenopausal period occur 12 times more often than in older men. This leads to death in 25% of cases and to long-term disability in 25-30%. Although it is not easy to predict which older women will develop osteoporosis, new methods for examining bones can measure bone density and prescribe treatment on time.

It is now known that hormone replacement therapy can prevent the development of osteoporosis in the initial stages.

Myocardial infarction and coronary heart disease. Before menopause, the risk of cardiovascular disease in women is significantly lower than in men of the same age. It is assumed that this is due to the influence of estrogens on the content of certain substances in the blood, which are responsible for removing cholesterol from the body. In the postmenopausal period, this protective effect is lost, and the risk of developing cardiovascular diseases increases sharply because the walls of small arteries become less elastic. The risk of cardiovascular disease can be reduced by exercise, appropriate diet, and hormone replacement therapy.

Diet and lifestyle

It is important to lead a healthy lifestyle, and it is also especially important to follow a diet during menopause.

Physical activity. Exercise keeps your heart and circulatory system in good condition and helps keep your bones strong and strong. Physically active people are usually more energetic, they are less likely to have bouts of angina pectoris and myocardial infarction, and if they do, then such patients recover more quickly. Any amount of exercise is better than nothing, however, an hour of intense walking, dancing, swimming or cycling at least three times a week will help keep your body in good shape. Physical activity should be diverse in order to strengthen the three areas of increased risk of bone fractures -

forearm, spine, and thigh. For example, swimming is good for the hands, walking for the spine and thighs. Exercise should be fun.

1. Walk short distances instead of using transport.

2. Try taking small daily walks.

3. Do not use the elevator; climb the stairs on foot.

4. Do not exercise if they are a burden to you.

Smoking and drinking. The health hazards of smoking are well known and difficult to overestimate. Smokers should completely get rid of this habit. If it is too difficult to give up smoking, then the maximum possible reduction in the number of cigarettes smoked will bring some benefit. Alcohol should not be consumed excessively, as abuse of it can cause obesity, a disease of the liver, brain, and heart. In addition, alcohol prevents the body from absorbing calcium ions, thereby increasing the risk of osteoporosis.

Diet and health. With age, both men and women tend to take more food than the body requires, which causes the appearance of excess weight. Often preference is given to convenience foods, which by no means always provide a balanced diet, which is necessary for a healthy diet. Food should contain balanced amounts of fats, carbohydrates, and proteins, as well as appropriate minerals and vitamins.

• Dairy products are rich in calcium, but some also contain a lot of fat. Nonfat and homemade cheeses in this sense are better than hard cheese, skim milk is better than whole, and unsweetened nonfat yogurt is better than its high-fat varieties.

• It is preferable to eat more fish, chicken, legumes, and nuts than red meat and eggs. All visible fat should be removed from the meat before cooking and, if possible, it is better to grill the meat than to fry it.

• A table rich in fats is one of the factors causing breast and colon cancer, while coarser foods with high fiber content are considered a means of preventing malignant tumors. Vegetables, fruits, unfinished cereals, and foods such as wholemeal bread and pasta are a good source of fiber.

• The recommended calcium intake for young people is 500 mg daily. This corresponds to approximately 0.5 liters of milk. Women over 60 are advised to consume twice as much calcium. The most affordable sources of calcium are dairy products, herbs and bony varieties of small fish. Calcium can also be obtained in the form of tablets if its intake into the body with products is insufficient. It is also important to remember that vitamin D is needed to absorb calcium; In the human body, the formation of vitamin D is facilitated by sunburn. Food sources of this vitamin are dairy and sour-milk products, fish oil and fortified varieties of margarine. However, remember that calcium alone does not cure osteoporosis and does not prevent it - this requires HRT.

• Foods rich in fats, especially animals, can lead to atherosclerosis. In this case, the lumen of the arteries narrows, which leads to an increase in blood pressure, cardiovascular diseases, and myocardial infarction. The risk of these complications in postmenopausal women increases when estrogen deficiency leads to changes in the metabolism and transport of cholesterol. Replenishment of estrogen in the form of HRT can correct the situation, however, in this case, it is more reasonable to adhere to the principles of a healthy diet.

Other Health Tips

Some women believe that as soon as they have stopped their periods, the risk of developing breast cancer or cervical cancer has disappeared. This is not so, and women should regularly, twice a year, undergo preventive examinations with their gynecologists to take a smear from the cervix. Of particular importance is the regular self-examination of the mammary glands, which, however, does not replace the usual medical examination. There is currently strong evidence that regular post-menopausal mammograms help early detection of breast cancer and reduce mortality from it. You should also regularly measure blood pressure. Any unexpected bleeding from the vagina is considered an abnormality, and if it occurs, you should definitely consult a doctor.

The causes of uterine bleeding in postmenopausal women are:

1. Dysfunctional bleeding (impaired ovarian function).

2. Pathological conditions associated with organ disease (endometrial adenocarcinoma, uterine fibroids, polyps, adenomyosis, hormone-active ovarian tumors, endometrial hyperplasia).

One of the first symptoms of the development of such serious conditions is spotting from the uterus. The key to your health is a timely request for professional help.

Therapeutic gymnastics with prolapse of the uterus

A small, hard wadding pillow always lies on the sofa. So at any time, going to rest, put a pillow under your hips and do some exercises. There is no need to lay a pillow under your head. Then the body will have a slope of 20–35 °.

Important exercise: squeeze the knees, squeeze the muscles of the perineum with force, retract the anus and stomach. Squeezed - inhale, relaxed - exhale. Still, the body is motionless, and you bend to one side and the other with effort, while the lateral abdominal muscles and the spine work.

Massage the lower abdomen. Lubricate your hands with any cream, you can use sunflower oil, put a pillow or roller under your hips, legs bent at the knees. Massage, knead well the perineum, pubis, appendages, lower abdomen towards the navel. Then pull the edge of the palm also towards the navel. It is necessary to strengthen the weakened muscles of the pelvic floor.

Muscles under such a load should receive good nutrition. In the morning you need to eat any nuts, peanuts, sunflower seeds, pumpkins.

Put on the floor a clean, in-line rug, roll the roller from an old sweater and lay on your back. Place the roller under the buttocks so that there is a slope: the head on the floor, and the buttocks on the roller. Straighten your legs, arms along the body.

1. Lift the left leg by 90 °, without bending the knees, lower it, now raise the right leg, lower it (6-7 times).

2. Together, raise the legs 90 °, without bending the knees, lower (6-7 times).

3. "Scissors" - 20-30 seconds.

4. "Bicycle" - 20-30 seconds.

5. Legs together, straight. Now left foot - to the side and rotate around the axis for 20-30

seconds. Then the right leg to the side and rotate around its axis for 20-30 seconds.

6. Legs together, lift without bending the knees, at the same time raise your hands so that the fingers touch the toes (6-7 times). Lower your legs.

7. Legs together, lift with your knees bent, tilt to the left and then to the right at the same time so that your back does not come off the floor (6-7 times).

8. Bend your legs at the knees, hands - under the buttocks, without taking your shoulders off the floor (6-7 times).

9. "Candle" - 20-30 seconds.

10. Remove the roller, do the "Top".

11. Lie down on the roller belly, legs straight, arms in front. At the same time, lift your arms

and legs above the floor for 20-30 seconds (6-7 times).

12. Get on all fours and bend your back up and down (6-7 times).

13. Standing on all fours, straighten the right leg, then the left (6-7 times).

14. Get up. Hold the chair with your left hand, the right leg to the side, wave (6-7 times). Now the other way.

15. Hold the chair with your left hand, and rotate around your axis with your right foot, now change your foot (6-7 times).

16. The Swallow.

You cannot jump and run. Do exercises every day on an empty stomach. Do not lift weights.

WHAT IS KETO DIET

The conversation of the keto diet plan has actually been continuous for numerous years, and throughout this duration, it has actually had the ability to collect lots of enthusiastic fans in weight-loss and females over the age of 50. In general terms, a keto diet plan and its versions are diet plans enriched in fats and proteins with an exceptionally low quantity of carbohydrate material (normally less than 10% of the overall quantity of macronutrients); with such diet plan, the body is required to make use of fats as fuel, given that glucose shops are quickly diminished.

For lots of, a ketogenic diet plan can be a really appropriate and efficient method to accomplish your objectives, whether it is developing muscle, burning fat, establishing strength signs, and so on. The ketogenic diet plan is utilized mainly for physical fitness and health functions, it can likewise be utilized as an anti-aging diet plan specifically in females over the age of 50.

In truth, there are not numerous distinctions. Numerous individuals think that such a dietary system ends up being maximally reliable when the body emerges into a state called "ketosis," and begins to manufacture ketones for subsequent energy generation (thus the name of the diet plan is "ketogenic"), and such a shift is possible just if one limitations carbohydrate consumption.

In the proposed guide, we will study in detail the physiological procedures that underlie the ketogenic diet plan, have a look at the current types/ alternatives of ketogenic diet plans, discover how to make your own diet plan and provide some basic suggestions on how to excite the cravings for low-carb foods. And, obviously, we will respond to the most typical concerns.

ketosis

As discussed previously, the ketogenic diet plan got its name due to the reality that the constraint of carb consumption attribute of this food system can put the body into a state of ketosis - a unique physiological state in which the concentration of ketone bodies boosts.

Ketone bodies are natural biomolecules soluble in liquid media that are manufactured in the liver from fats while decreasing food consumption (specifically carb). After being transferred to extrahepatic tissues, these biomolecules can be utilized as an energy source.

In percentages, ketone bodies are continuously manufactured in the body, however, generally, the concentration of ketones is so low that they are not discovered in the analysis of urine. When the level of ketone bodies in the blood increases (a condition understood as ketonemia), they start to be excreted in the urine (the so-called ketonuria); ketonemia and ketonuria are taken together suggest the shift of the body to a state of ketosis.

The objective of a ketogenic diet plan is to move the body to a state of food ketosis (not to be puzzled with pathological ketosis), which eventually directs the metabolic process to the usage of fatty acids and ketone bodies as the primary source of energy.

ketogenic diet options

There are 3 primary choices for a ketogenic diet plan: a basic ketogenic diet plan (SKD), a cyclic ketogenic diet plan (CKD), and a targeted ketogenic diet plan (TKD). The kind of diet plan you require is picked entirely by experimentation and is mainly identified by top priority objectives (in more information listed below).

A standard ketogenic diet

This is the simplest form of a keto diet. It is the most common diet that we all have been discussing. I will not go into details about this type of keto diet at the moment because this type will become clear to you in a short while.

A cyclic ketogenic diet

What exactly is Cyclical Ketogenic Diet?

The basic or standard keto diet plan is a high fat, low carbohydrate, moderate protein diet plan. It normally includes consuming in between 5 - 10% of your calories from carbohydrates (20 - 50 grams a day) with 60% or more of the staying calories from fat.

The objective of limiting carbs is to reach a metabolic state called ketosis, where the body starts to burn fat instead of sugar for its fuel source.

The CKD includes turning in between a stringent low carbohydrate keto diet plan and a greater carbohydrate diet plan 1 - 2 days a week. It's a more versatile technique for a keto diet plan.

The versatility appears enticing, the cyclic keto diet plan isn't for everybody. It's not perfect for those utilizing the keto diet plan to handle health conditions, control blood glucose levels, or weight reduction. Increasing carbohydrates will slow your development if those are your objectives.

Those seeking to enhance workout or sports efficiency might discover the CKD appealing as it uses versatility while still taking advantage of a low carbohydrate way of life.

Something to keep in mind about the cyclic keto diet plan is that there is no research study behind this dieting approach.

The cyclic keto diet plan was created due to the fact that numerous professional athletes carry out much better with increased carb consumption, however, they still desired the many advantages that keto needs to provide. With this approach, professional athletes can get the very best of both worlds.

Cyclical Keto Diet or Standard Keto Diet

The primary distinction in between CKD and the basic ketogenic diet plan is the variety of carbohydrates you're taking in.

On a basic keto diet plan, you would never ever increase your carbohydrate consumption beyond 20 - 50 grams a day.

On a CKD, you consume keto 5 - 6 days a week, then increase your carbohydrates 1 - 2 days a week. The greater carbohydrate days are your refeeding days.

Throughout your refeeding days, you'll be bumped out of ketosis. You must be able to get back to ketosis within a couple of days of going back to low carbohydrate consumption if you've been on keto for a while. Your body will come utilized to changing from these 2 fuel sources effectively with mindful meal fasting, workout, and preparation.

How to do a Cyclical Keto Diet?

There are no agreed-upon guidelines for precisely how to do a cyclic keto diet plan. This diet plan needs some experimentation to discover the very best approach that assists you to attain your physical fitness objectives.

One method to get going is to consume a rigorous keto diet plan for 6 days. You initially require to enter into ketosis to begin the cycle.

We've put together a fast no-brainer guide if you require a refresher or some brand-new concepts for your keto diet plan grocery list. The very best method to begin your keto diet plan is by meal remaining and prepping on top of your food alternatives to prevent falling under yearnings.

Goal to keep your carbohydrate consumption between 20 - 50 grams a day and consume a lot of healthy fats. On the 7th day, increase your carbohydrate consumption and limit your fat consumption. Keep protein the exact same throughout.

Is Cyclic Keto Right for You?

In theory, cyclic keto takes the very best of both worlds of keto and high carbohydrate consumption. It utilizes carbohydrates for muscle-building and hormone advantages while enhancing development hormonal agent with ketosis. It might likewise appear interesting to have the ability to sometimes bump up your carbohydrate consumption.

Cyclic keto is most likely not the perfect diet plan for the typical individual. It would just be suggested for professional athletes who have actually experienced declines in efficiency while consuming keto. It might be one approach to enhance efficiency and body structure, although there is no research study to support these claims.

For the majority of women over 50 who simply wish to reduce weight and develop a little bit of muscle, there is a lot of research study behind the advantages of a basic keto diet plan to fulfill those objectives.

The targeted ketogenic diet

This resembles the standard ketogenic diet plan (SKD) in regards to your diet strategy most the time-- Both are high fat, low carbohydrate diet plans. The macronutrient breakdowns of TKD and SKD are comparable, with 5 - 10% of calories originating from carbohydrates, 60 - 80% from fat, and the rest from protein. The primary distinction in between targeted and basic keto is that on targeted keto carbohydrate consumption modifications. On the basic keto diet plan, you constantly keep your carbohydrates low. On the targeted keto diet plan, you would consume additional carbohydrates prior to, throughout, or after an exercise. On exercise days, your carbohydrate macros may increase a little, and your fat macros would reduce. Your only constant here is your protein consumption-- it must constantly stay the exact same to support lean muscle development.

Targeted Ketogenic Diet or Cyclical Ketogenic Diet

The targeted keto diet plan might appear comparable to the cyclical keto diet plan (CKD) if you're familiar with the various variations of ketogenic dieting. Both include carbohydrate biking, briefly slipping out of ketosis for the advantage of enhanced workout efficiency.

When you consume them, the primary distinction between targeted and cyclic keto is the number of carbohydrates you consume and.

On a cyclical ketogenic diet plan, you turn your fat and carbohydrate macros a couple of days a week. This might indicate you're consuming 80% carbohydrates and just 5 - 10% fat on high carbohydrate days.

With TKD, you would just bump up your carbohydrates just around your high-intensity exercises-- not for the entire day. On a TKD, you're most likely to consume fewer carbohydrates in general compared to CKD.

Advantages of the Targeted Keto Diet

Targeted keto likely has lots of advantages compared to the basic ketogenic diet plan, such as weight-loss, cravings control, and enhanced brainpower.

Let's take a better take a look at 2 other reasons that individuals might try out TKD.

Improved Exercise Performance

The primary advantage of TKD over the basic keto diet plan is that it might enhance workout efficiency. Consuming carbohydrates around your exercises fill your muscle glycogen shops, which are easily utilized by the body to offer an energy increase throughout the workout, particularly for endurance occasions.

Increased Muscle Mass

Like cyclic keto, targeted keto might likewise assist increase lean muscle mass. The basic keto diet plan can assist increase muscle by itself, however, if you do not see the outcomes you desire, it might be because of low insulin levels.

Insulin is a muscle-building hormonal agent. In theory, comparable to cyclic keto, increasing your insulin levels pre-workout offers your muscles additional glucose to burn, which will enhance efficiency and assist you to develop more muscle.

Bumping up your carbohydrate consumption does not simply affect insulin-- it can likewise customize other hormonal agents that assist construct muscle. Another hormonal agent called development hormonal agent is required for bodybuilding and weight reduction.

Development hormonal agent is low when insulin is raised. When you return into ketosis after your exercise, and your insulin levels drop once again, your development hormonal agent will increase.

Sometimes surging your insulin will assist you to get the very best of both worlds and optimize muscle development and workout efficiency.

It's essential to restate that these proposed advantages are all theoretical based upon a basic understanding of human physiology.

There are no research studies that have actually assessed the best dosage of carbohydrates, perfect timing, or how targeted keto is finest used-- if you wish to give it a try, you will need to be your own guinea pig.

Who is the Targeted Keto Diet For?

The targeted keto diet plan was developed for sophisticated keto dieters and professional athletes who might discover their sports efficiency suffers on the basic ketogenic diet plan. This diet strategy is best for individuals who practice high-intensity workouts such as expert athletes, runners, bodybuilders, or Crossfit professional athletes.

The increased carb consumption around exercises will assist you to minimize tiredness and support blood glucose levels. It's not for every type of exercise.

There is some proof that recommends that carbohydrate re-feeding might do little to enhance efficiency throughout strength exercises. This might be since weight lifting does not consume a great deal of glycogen, so the muscles aren't starving for additional carbohydrates.

Carbs on Targeted Keto Diet

A targeted keto diet plan is relatively comparable to a basic keto diet plan. The macronutrient breakdown would be as follows:

Fat: 60 - 80%.

Protein: 20 - 30%.

Carbohydrates: 5 - 10%.

Foods consisted of a targeted keto diet plan are:

Healthy fats: olive oil, avocados, nuts, coconut oil, MCT oil, butter.

Protein: chicken, fish, beef, lamb, eggs, cheese.

Low carb veggies.

Little portions of nuts and berries.

The list above is what you would consume the majority of the time while following the low carbohydrate part of the diet plan.

Prior to, throughout, or after your exercise, you wish to consume in between 15 - 50 grams of fast-absorbing carbohydrates. Fast-absorbing carbohydrates normally do not include a substantial quantity of fiber, fat, or protein.

A couple of alternatives for fast-acting carbohydrates consist of:

White rice.

Spud.

White bread.

Crackers.

Glucose shot.

Sports beverages like Gatorade.

Energy gummi.

Hard candy.

Dextrose powder.

It's advised that foods high in fructose, like fruit juice or soda, need to be prevented on a TKD since fructose is not easily utilized for energy by the muscles like glucose is.

Fructose goes straight to the liver to be kept as glycogen, so it will not assist you to increase your efficiency.

Preparation Your Targeted Keto Diet Based On Your Goal.

How you time your exercise carbohydrates and the number of carbohydrates you take in will depend upon your individual objectives, however here are some basic standards.

Enhanced Performance During a Workout (less than 1 hour).

Consume 15 - 50 grams of fast-acting carbohydrates about thirty minutes prior to your work out.

If your exercise is less than 45 minutes, think about consuming on the low end of this variety of the advised carbohydrates, or you will not have the ability to burn all the carbohydrates throughout your workout. Return to consuming keto right away after an exercise.

Long Endurance Workout (over 1 hour or in severe hot or cold).

Consume 15 - 50 grams of fast-acting carbohydrates 30 minutes prior to your exercise.

Consume 6 - 12 ounces of a sports drink or a gel with at least a 6% carbohydrate concentration every 30 minutes. Resume typical keto consumption after the exercise.

Increase in General Exercise Performance.

To typically raise your workout efficiency and take full advantage of muscle gain, consume 15 - 50 grams of fast-acting carbohydrates 30 minutes pre-workout.

Post-workout, consume another 15 - 50 grams of carbohydrates. This will permit you to enhance the post-workout insulin spike required for bodybuilding.

These are simply standards of where to begin for your targeted keto diet plan. Discovering your perfect variety of carbohydrates and timing will take experimentation prior to you begin to see the gains from this procedure.

How Does a Targeted Keto Diet Impact Ketosis?

Whenever you increase your carbohydrate consumption you momentarily knock yourself out of ketosis. If you are disciplined and fat-adapted, you ought to be back into ketosis within a couple of hours.

Because you're timing the carbohydrates around your exercise, your body needs to easily take in the excess glucose to sustain your muscles.

This suggests, after an especially difficult exercise, your blood glucose levels will not remain high for long. How rapidly your blood sugar level and insulin levels go back to regular depends upon the kind of exercise and how delicate you are to insulin.

There are a couple of methods you can return into ketosis much faster.

Attempt doing some light to moderate-intensity steady-state cardio after your exercise. A light exercise keeps your body in fat-burning mode, which will assist it to begin burning ketones once again.

You can include premium MCT oil to your routine. MCTs rapidly increase the number of ketones in your body, assisting you to return into ketosis much faster. You can explore utilizing MCT oil prior to or after your exercise to enhance energy and boost ketones.

These techniques might assist you to get back into ketosis much faster, how rapidly this takes place depends on lots of elements beyond your control. The finest thing you can do is just consume a typical keto diet plan once again as quickly as your exercise is over.

Keto option to adopt

Evaluate how your body responds to changes in diet, how your performance changes, and how energetic you are. After that, it will be easier to decide which diet to use

Many factors will influence your choice of diet type. It is recommended to start with the "break-in period" using a standard ketogenic diet. In a few weeks of such a break-in, you will be able to evaluate how the body reacts to a change in diet, how your physical performance changes, and how energetic you are. After that, it will be easier for you to decide which diet should be used over a long distance.

You may also have doubts about which option is best for losing weight, and which is ideal for gaining muscle mass. It must be said that if the total energy value of your diet meets the objectives, the ketogenic diet option will not become a key factor on the way to achieving the goal. You may come across the opinion that CKD or TKD is better suited for people who want to gain muscle mass since carbohydrates save protein and stimulate insulin secretion, and standard keto diet will be an ideal choice for those who want to lose weight since insulin synthesis will be relatively low. However, these short-term fluctuations in insulin secretion over a long distance will not be a decisive factor, in

HOW TO MAKE YOUR OWN KETO DIET

In this section, we will talk about how to determine the body's needs for energy and macronutrients, these figures will become your basic guidelines in compiling the ACS diet. People who make the choice in favor of CKD or TKD will also have to use basic calculations for ACS, but with minor adjustments, which I will discuss later.

In general, we can say that everyone who wants to lose weight should adhere to the golden rule of a daily deficit of 500 calories, and those who want to gain muscle mass must achieve an excess of the same 500 calories. However, this is too crude a generalization without taking into account physiological characteristics and other factors. In addition, if you choose for yourself CKD, you will most likely have to adjust the calorie intake for one week.

Here is an example of how to calculate the consumption of macronutrients for ACS:

Determine energy requirements using a daily calorie calculator;

Daily protein requirement 2 g / kg dry weight: 150 g per day

The need for carbohydrates 0.2-0.4 g / kg dry weight: 15-30 g per day (hereinafter in the calculations we proceed from 30 g)

Since 1 g of protein and carbohydrates contain 4 calories, we have (150 + 30) x 4: 720 calories from proteins and carbohydrates

We get that this person should receive 1280 calories with fats (2000 - 720), and since there are 9 calories in one gram of fat, he should eat about 142 (1280 divided by 9) grams of fat daily.

Thus, in total, the daily diet of this person will be 150 grams of protein, 30 grams of carbohydrates and 142 grams of fat. Distribute this amount between meals.

As a side bonus here is an example of a 3 days meal plan

	Squirrels	Carbohydrates	Fats
1st meal	50 g	10 g	48 g
2nd meal	50 g	10 g	47 g
3rd meal	50 g	10 g	47 g

As a side bonus here is an example of a 5-meal meal plan:

	Squirrels	Carbohydrates	Fats
1st meal	30 g	5 g	29 g
2nd meal	30 g	5 g	29 g
3rd meal	30 g	5 g	28 g
4th meal	30 g	5 g	28 g
5th meal	30 g	5 g	28 g

SELECTING THE RIGHT FOOD ON KETO DIET

There are no strict rules in the ketogenic diet, as there are no permitted or prohibited foods. Many are sure that the main sources of starch and sugar should not be included in the diet since this will prevent the metabolism from switching to ketosis, but in negligible amounts, such products are unlikely to become an obstacle, especially for large people.

The following foods are a good choice for a ketogenic diet:

- Any kind of protein from an animal's origin (especially red meat)
- Eggs (whole or protein only)
- Fatty dairy products such as cheese, cream, butter, etc.

- Oils, preferably vegetable, peanuts, flax seeds, macadamia, olives and certain varieties of coconut

- Nuts and Nut Pastes

Fibrous vegetables, especially greens, lettuce, broccoli, celery, etc.

During the consumption of the ketogenic diet, do not limit yourself and include more sources of starch and sugars, such as fruits, in your diet.

CKD PLANNING FOR WOMEN OVER 50

Now let's see how you should integrate carbohydrates into the cyclic version of the ketogenic diet when you are over the age of.

Those women over the age of 50 who choose CKD should start with carbohydrate consumption once a week, and then, as necessary, change the time interval between loading days in accordance with their individual needs. Get ready for the fact that you will have to conduct a lot of experiments, during which you will evaluate how much carbohydrates you ate on a busy day, and how you feel in the following days.

The main thing to keep in mind when consuming carbohydrates is to reduce fat intake; do not continue to eat fat in large portions on initial days. But leave the protein intake at the same level (or even increase to maintain the total calorie content).

Using the requirements for the macronutrients of the previously mentioned 75-kg person, we give the basic recommendations regarding the configuration of CKD with one consumption day, depending on the individual sensitivity to insulin/tolerance to carbohydrates:

The need for protein in **women over 50**2 g / kg dry weight: 150 g / day

With low sensitivity to insulin in women over 50 - we calculate the consumption of carbohydrates based on the calculation of 2-3 g per kg of dry weight

With normal sensitivity to insulin in **women over 50**- we calculate the consumption of carbohydrates based on the calculation of 4-5 g per kg of dry weight

With high sensitivity to insulin in women over 50 - we calculate the consumption of carbohydrates based on the calculation of 6-7 g per kg of dry weight

Now, as before, we simply count the remaining calories, divide by 9 and get the grams of fat that you need to get on days loaded with carbohydrates

An example of CKD for people with normal sensitivity to insulin and a dry body weight of 75 kg, adhering to a restrictive diet of 2000 calories:

Monday - **Saturday**: nutrient intake should be consistent with previously calculated requirements for ACS

Sunday (carbohydrate consumption day, 2500 calories) - 150 g protein / 300 g carbohydrates / 78 g fat

TKD PLANNING FOR WOMEN OVER 50

Now let's see how to integrate carbohydrates into the targeted version of the ketogenic diet for women over the age of 50.

As in the case of CKD, when starting TKD, first evaluate how your body reacts to certain amounts of carbohydrates, and determine for yourself the optimal time for their intake. Remember, observing TKD, you should take a sufficient amount of carbohydrates for optimal performance, but not abuse them. CKD suggests periods of glycogen replenishment, while TKD aims only at a short-term increase in energy and performance.

Therefore, if an athlete is training intensively 5 days a week, he must consume carbohydrates before and/or after training on these training days. In the remaining days, nutrient intake should be consistent with the estimates for SKD.

Calculation of nutrient requirements during TCD, in fact, is no different from SKD, we only add carbohydrates to the "near-training" meal on training days. As an illustration of how to plan a training intake of carbohydrates for TCD, we suggest using the recommendations for the same 75 kg athlete who is in the drying phase, receives 2000 calories daily and has a certain sensitivity to insulin/carbohydrate tolerance:

The need for protein in women over 50 2 g / kg dry weight: 150 g / day

With low sensitivity to insulin in women over 50 - add 0.5 g of carbohydrates per 1 kg of dry weight to the "near-training" meal

With normal sensitivity to insulin in women over 50- add 0.75 g of carbohydrates per 1 kg of dry weight to the "near-training" meal

With high sensitivity to insulin in women over 50 - add 1 g of carbohydrates per 1 kg of dry weight to the "near-training" meal

Now we subtract the "extra" calories from carbohydrates and protein from the daily energy requirement and get the missing calories from fats (everything is as before).

The "near-training" meal precedes the training session or follows after it. This means that you can arbitrarily distribute the "extra" carbohydrates, as long as they are all eaten within the training window. In general, it is recommended that you simply divide the total amount in half and eat them before and after your workout.

An example of a diet with TCD with five meals for women over 50 and with 75 kg

of dry weight and high sensitivity to insulin, which is on a 3000-calorie diet per weight:

	Squirrels	Carbohydrates	Fats
1st meal (before training)	30 g	40 g	20 g
2nd meal (after training)	30 g	35 g	20 g
3rd meal	30 g	10 g	30 g
4th meal	30 g	10 g	30 g
5th meal	30 g	10 g	30 g

THE ROLE OF SATURATED FATS IN WOMEN OVER 50 AND ON A KETOGENIC DIET

Starting a ketogenic diet will inevitably lead to an increase in the proportion of saturated fats in your diet, but this does not mean that you should completely rely on saturated fats and ignore the consumption of polyunsaturated fats.

Around how much-saturated fat in a ketogenic diet is considered excessive, lively discussions are underway. Many people who have tried a ketogenic diet insist on impressive portions of foods such as butter, fatty red meat, fatty dairy products, etc.

Saturated fats are related to the production of sex hormones (androgens) in the body of men, and therefore a sharp reduction in their consumption can hardly be called a good idea. However, the constant abuse of saturated fats can lead to an increase in insulin resistance and other metabolic disorders, so filling the body with these nutrients is also not part of our plans. This is a bit different for women over 50. It is necessary to consume saturated fat when you are over the age of 50. This will strengthen your body and freshen your skin. But it has nothing to do with your hormones.

In my opinion, against the background of a ketogenic diet, you can raise the proportion of saturated fats in the diet to 20-30% of the total amount of fats without any fears. That is, if a person receives 150 g of fat daily with food, he should try to limit the amount of saturated fat to 30-45 grams per day.

We have long been told that eating fatty foods makes us fat and contributes to the development of cardiovascular diseases. But it's time to debunk this myth! More and more modern studies are proving that consuming the right types of dietary fat provides tremendous health benefits and helps to lose those extra pounds in women over 50. That's right - fats are good for our bodies!

The need for fats

Forget everything that you heard or read about fatty foods that make you fat. The human body needs natural fats, which is why many of them are called "essential fatty acids. " The word "irreplaceable" means that the body requires them for various processes, but cannot produce them on its own. That's why we need to get essential fatty acids from our diet.

Fats are useful because they perform many important functions for our health. Here are just a few of them:

- Improve the absorption of fat-soluble vitamins,
- Optimize metabolism
- Provide a supply of energy in the body,
- Protect the body from the cold,
- Support healthy skin, hair, and nails,
- Help the body absorb nutrients
- Contribute to the proper functioning of nerves, brain, and heart.

As you can see, fats in foods are not something "scary", on the contrary, they are vital for a person to maintain health and well-being. This applies equally to both unsaturated fats (systemic) and saturated fats. Modern scientists have refuted the old recommendations regarding nutrition, as they have not found any scientifically based connection between the intake of saturated fats and the increased risk of heart disease.

Here are some reasons why fats are good for your diet

People do not grow fat from fat but from sugar. The media made us think of fats as "killers," causing obesity, disease, and miserable death. Yes, we were thoroughly brainwashed and made to fear and hate any fats. Instead, with the help of advertising, food corporations slipped us sugar: in any form, in any wrapper, at any age. And this despite the fact that not fats, namely refined sugar and processed carbohydrates, lead to almost instant unhealthy weight gain. Sugar and simple carbohydrates break down into simple sugars during digestion. All this excess sugar in the blood causes insulin insensitivity. It is usually difficult for a person to burn all the sugar that she consumes at once. As a result, the body accumulates excess sugar in the form of fat, and all excess insulin in the blood leads to insulin resistance and metabolic disorder. Only a diet high in fiber will help protect against excessive spikes in blood glucose (sugar) levels.

If fats are removed from any food, something else needs to be added to it to give it a pleasant taste and to make the eater feel full. This "something else" is often hidden sugar. Low-fat diet foods containing sugar and starch are bad for heart health. A 2007 study found that almost 75% of patients hospitalized with a heart attack had normal cholesterol. But they had elevated blood sugar, prediabetes or type 2 diabetes. We conclude - pay attention to the label and do not fall for the inscription "low fat"!

Unlike sugars, fats have a complex chemical structure. All sugars, natural or artificial, cause the same harm to the body. The structure of sugar is simple, so it is quickly absorbed, and its level in the blood is able to rise and fall sharply.

Unlike sugar, the structure of fats is complex. There are about forty different fatty acids, so their numerous combinations are very common. Fatty acids are made up of long chains of carbon atoms bonded to oxygen atoms and two hydrogen atoms. Saturated, monounsaturated, polyunsaturated, and even trans fats exist. Although not all of them are beneficial to humans, they go through a more complex digestion process than sugar. And this is crucial for maintaining satiety and a healthy metabolism.

Fats are indispensable for the proper functioning of the brain and nervous system in women over the age of 50. The brain is 60% fat, of which most are docosahexaenoic acid (DHA) or omega-3 fats. Research has linked omega-3 fatty acid deficiencies to a variety of mental disorders, including depression, anxiety, bipolar disorder, and schizophrenia. Omega-3 fatty acids help support the nervous, communicative, and protective functions of the body.

Fats contribute to weight loss. The presence of fat in the diet, while reducing carbohydrate intake, maybe the secret to losing weight. We recommend a diet low in simple carbohydrates and high in fat, which helps improve insulin sensitivity and lose weight. Healthy fats can mobilize reserves of subcutaneous fat, using them as an energy source. As a result, improved insulin function provides satiety and helps control appetite. Eat foods rich in good fats and you will feel full faster and longer. And since fats are absorbed much more slowly compared to carbohydrates, you will eat smaller portions and will not feel hungry soon after eating.

Fats are critical to sexual health. Fats are the building blocks for cell membranes, but they are also important for hormonal health. Our sex hormones - testosterone, estrogen, progesterone - all are based on cholesterol. Reducing dietary fat intake may increase the risk of hormonal diseases such as hypothyroidism, menstrual irregularities in women, and low testosterone in men.

Fats help build strong bones. Even if you are using nutritional supplements to strengthen bones, hoping that this will help reduce the risk of osteoporosis and arthritis in the future, you will need fats for this. This is due to the fact that the vitamins A, D, E and K necessary for bone formation are only fat-soluble. This means that they are transported and absorbed using dietary fats. Fats are essential for calcium metabolism. This mineral cannot be effectively incorporated into bone tissue without fats!

Misconception regarding saturated fats. There is no reason to be afraid of saturated fats. Studies show that there is no correlation between saturated fats and heart disease. However, not all saturated fats are formed in the same way. The greasy cheeseburger from the nearest fast food restaurant does not contain as much saturated heart fats as a tablespoon of coconut oil. Therefore, you should not classify all saturated fats as equally healthy.

We need more omega-3 fats! A fanatical obsession with "good" fats, namely polyunsaturated fats, can do more harm than good. This is due to the fact that polyunsaturated fats cover both beneficial omega-3s and those that cause inflammatory processes, omega-6s. Of course, we need both types of these fats. But the researchers found that a typical Western diet has a ratio of 15: 1-

16.7: 1 (omega-6: omega-3), which indicates a deficiency of omega-3 fatty acids. We consume excess omega-6 fatty acids compared to the diet humans evolved on. Try to include more omega-3 rich foods in your diet to optimize your healthy diet (linseed oil, chia oil, fish oil).

Limit the intake of trans fats! It is better to avoid the use of trans fats from burned vegetable oils. Competent nutritionists, guided by the results of recent studies, advise limiting to a minimum in your diet any refined oils and trans fats, such as margarine contained in baked goods because they are associated with chronic age-related diseases.

Eat the right fats

Now that we have found out why fats are good for women over 50, let's talk about how to eat right. According to the recommendations of the American Heart Association, the best ratio of saturated, monounsaturated and polyunsaturated fats in a healthy diet should be 6: 4: 1. There is evidence that increased consumption of polyunsaturated fats (up to 15 percent daily calories) instead of saturated fats can reduce the risk of heart disease.

List of healthy fats:

- High-quality saturated fats from sources such as coconut oil, ghee, and animal fats consumed with meat.

- High-quality monounsaturated fats from sources such as peanut butter, sesame oil, and olive oil. Always choose cold-pressed oil; never buy cheaper thermally or chemically extracted oil.

You can also find high-quality fats in nature. Avocados and nuts are excellent sources of monounsaturated fats. Flax, sunflower, pumpkin, chia seeds, walnuts, and oily fish such as salmon, mackerel, herring, tuna, and trout are all good sources of polyunsaturated fats rich in omega-3s.

KETONES AND KETOSIS FOR WOMEN OVER THE AGE OF 50

Ketosis is a metabolic state that is set off when the body has actually consumed its primary energy source: glucose (or sugar). When this occurs, your body breaks down fat and transforms it into ketones, which then takes control of as your main kind of fuel.

Your body shops glucose in the kind of glycogen in the liver and muscles. Getting into a ketosis state will vary by private according to one's age, metabolic process, workout level, and macronutrient (fat, carbohydrate, and protein) consumption.

Getting Into Ketosis

Accomplishing ketosis needs a diet plan low in carbs and high in fat, with a moderate quantity of protein. This implies you'll be consuming around:

Fats: 60-80%.

Proteins: 15-30%.

Carbohydrates: 5-10%.

Net carbohydrates can be computed by taking a food's overall quantity of carbs and deducting its fiber material. Computing net carbohydrates motivate you to consume more fiber-rich whole foods, which can be more difficult to get on a keto or low-carb diet plan.

The majority of the carbohydrates you eliminated will be changed with fats. This consists of foods like; avocados, olives, MCT Oil, additional virgin olive and coconut oil, grass-fed butter and full-fat dairy.

As soon as you've substantially reduced your carbohydrates to under 50 grams, accomplishing ketosis can frequently take just 2-4 days, though it might take a week or longer for some individuals.

Remaining in ketosis is identified by the level of ketones in your blood. Particularly, when you've reached a limit of a minimum of 0.5 mmol/L of the ketone beta-hydroxybutyrate (BHB), your body is thought about to be in ketosis.

The fastest way to get into Ketosis

Cut carbohydrates. As talked about above, in order to get into Ketosis you need to cut carbohydrates. You can't out work out carbohydrate consumption, it begins constantly begins here.

Fasting: Going without food is the best method for ketosis, however, this does not indicate you need to starve yourself. Periodic fasting, which includes short-term fasts, will assist diminish those glycogen shops quicker to reach ketosis, often within simply 24 hours.

Taking In Coconut and/or MCT Oil: Research recommends that fat sources consisting of medium-chain triglycerides (MCTs), like coconut oil, can assist you to reach ketosis faster and assist you to sustain it. One research study discovered that a diet plan high in MCTs permitted for more carb consumption (upwards of 20% of calories), while still staying in ketosis.

Increasing Your Physical Activity: Exercising likewise assists diminish your glycogen shops, and it might even increase the production of ketones. Exercising while fasting might get you into ketosis even quicker.

Bear in mind your energy level, water intake, and mineral intake. Do not press yourself too hard, low strength workout is generally a much better alternative when you're making the switch to keto. Many individuals at first experience tiredness and low energy as their bodies adjust from utilizing glucose to ketones as fuel.

Taking Exogenous Ketones: These are dietary supplements that increase ketone levels in the blood. They likewise might assist to cause ketosis which we'll go over later on.

Take a Long Walk. This will assist you to shift to Ketosis, without exaggerating it.

Purchase a Ketone screening package. Urine strips aren't terrific indications, if you're stressed over the speed in which you accomplish ketosis you ought to actually have a precise method to determine it. This is an inexpensive, and reliable choice.

This isn't straight going to assist you to get into Ketosis much faster however it's going to make things a lot simpler. Guarantee you remain hydrated when transitioning to ketosis.

Take an Electrolyte Supplement. You'll likewise be flushing out crucial minerals when you're flushing out water. Taking an electrolyte ketone supplement will assist you to remain hydrated.

Types Of Ketones.

Ketones are acid spin-offs made by your liver when it breaks down fat-- both the fat you consume and the fat currently saved in your body-- for energy. There are 3 types of ketones (or ketone bodies):.

When fats are broken down, acetoacetate (AcAc) is the very first ketone produced. It then forms another kind of ketone, beta-hydroxybutyrate (BHB).

Beta-hydroxybutyrate (BHB) is the most effective and plentiful ketone produced in the body. This is why most ketone supplements, called exogenous ketones, are made with BHB.

Acetone is a by-product of AcAc, and it can trigger a fruity odor on your breath when your body remains in ketosis.

How to track Ketones.

To examine that your body remains in ketosis, you can determine ketone levels in your blood, breath, and urine.

Ketone urine strips are the least expensive and most convenient to utilize, however likewise the least precise since its determining the ketones that your body is eliminating, not utilizing.

A breathalyzer, which discovers acetone levels in your breath, is somewhat more trusted.

The finest tool for tracking your ketone levels is a blood ketone meter, which evaluates for blood levels of BHB. You can choose one up off amazon for $30.

How to know you are in Ketosis.

Aside from tracking ketones, you can likewise evaluate how you are feeling to identify whether your body remains in ketosis.

- Some individuals might experience the "keto influenza", which can last for simply a couple of days or as much as a couple of weeks. This generally consists of a group of signs, consisting of headache, queasiness, tiredness, sleeping disorders, irregularity, and irritation. Ensuring you remain consuming and hydrated lots of electrolytes can assist treat these signs quicker.

Other normal symptoms and signs to keep an eye out for, consist of:

- Increased thirst and more regular urination.
- " Keto breath" or fruity-smelling breath.
- Dry mouth.
- A decline in cravings.
- Weight reduction.
- Preliminary weak point and tiredness (this must ultimately decrease).
- Preliminary sleep disturbances (this need to likewise diminish).
- Increased energy, psychological clearness, and focus.

Exogenous Ketones

Endogenous ketones are produced internally in your liver, while exogenous ketones can be taken externally as a dietary supplement. Exogenous ketones include BHB considering that it's the most plentiful and effective in the body, and due to the fact that AcAc is not chemically steady adequate to be utilized. Supplements are offered in 2 primary types:

- Ketone salts: The most typical kind of exogenous ketones on the marketplace, these include BHB that is bound to salt, like calcium, salt, or potassium.

- Ketone esters: These ketones are integrated with alcohol and are frequently utilized in the research study.

Research study has actually revealed that exogenous ketones will increase blood ketone levels-- practically instantly-- and assist cause ketosis. This might be particularly efficient for those who wish to profit from ketosis without always following a stringent keto diet plan.

Advantages of Ketosis.

There's a growing quantity of research study concentrated on the possible advantages of keto and low-carb diet plans, and a lot of the outcomes are appealing. Keeping a stable state of ketosis can reduce hunger, result in weight-loss, reverse diabetes signs, increase brain function, and even possibly enhance the lives of those with Alzheimer's illness, Parkinson's illness, Multiple Sclerosis (MS), and cancer. Let's dig more into the research study.

Weight reduction.

Weight-loss from ketosis is triggered by a couple of various systems. Lots of individuals following a ketogenic diet plan will eventually consume fewer calories. Fats and proteins are even more pleasing and filling than carbs, so you might merely consume less.

There's likely more to it than the "calories in, calories out" theory. Many research studies have actually discovered that a low-carb keto diet plan results in more weight loss than other diet plans, even when the calorie consumption is equivalent. Simply see this one, which discovered that individuals on a keto diet plan lost 2.2 times more weight than those on a low-calorie, low-fat diet plan.

Part of this might be credited to hunger suppression. Remaining in ketosis can impact the hormonal agents connected to cravings and satiety, which suggests you might observe a decline in hunger. When on a ketogenic diet plan, this meta-analysis of different research studies concluded that ketosis appears to be the primary factor individuals feel less starving and more pleased.

This research study discovered that individuals on a ketogenic diet plan for 8 weeks lost an average of 13% of their body weight. Those who stayed in ketosis after the 8 weeks had lower levels of ghrelin (the "cravings hormonal agent") versus individuals no longer in ketosis. Another research study checked to make use of exogenous ketones and discovered that they likewise assisted reduce hunger by decreasing ghrelin levels in individuals.

Much more so, ketosis can likewise result in higher weight loss by increasing the quantity of fat you burn, whether you're exercising or just unwinding on the sofa.

Reduced Blood Sugar and Reversal of Diabetes.

Unlike glucose, ketones do not trigger blood sugar level variations. This is substantial for those with high blood glucose or anybody detected with pre-diabetes, diabetes, or metabolic syndrome.

In this research study of 28 clients with type 2 diabetes, a keto diet plan enhanced glycemic control-- a lot so that most of the individuals had the ability to terminate or considerably lower their use of diabetes medications.

Ketogenic diet plans are likewise associated with low insulin levels and enhanced insulin level of sensitivity, which can considerably enhance signs of type 2 diabetes.

Prospective Improvements in Alzheimer's, Parkinson's, Multiple Sclerosis, and Cancer.

Ketones, especially BHB, can help in reducing swelling and oxidative tension, both of which are connected with persistent conditions like diabetes and heart disease, along with Alzheimer's, Parkinson's, Multiple Sclerosis (MS), and cancer.

Early research study on ketosis and Alzheimer's is motivating, including this research study that reported substantial enhancements in memory, language, and attention for Alzheimer's clients who followed a stringent keto diet plan for four months. There might likewise be a great factor for consuming more coconut oil, as its fats might play a prospective function in dealing with and avoiding Alzheimer's.

These findings could be connected to ketosis' function in supporting blood glucose. Some scientists have actually described Alzheimer's as "type 3 diabetes," and have actually discovered that stabilizing your blood glucose can considerably decrease your danger of Alzheimer's.

Ketosis might likewise be helpful for different neurological conditions, like Parkinson's, as displayed in this research study, which reported considerable enhancements in motor and non-motor signs for those who kept ketosis for 8 weeks. There are likewise a couple of preliminary studies that reveal a ketogenic diet plan might enhance the lifestyle in those with MS.

On an even bigger scale, keto diet plans might play a significant function in cancer treatment. Research study has actually revealed that ketosis has the possibility to decrease tumor development, boost the efficiency of chemotherapy, and enhance the state of mind and sleep in clients with innovative cancer.

Durability.

Currently, the best anti-aging tool most researchers can settle on is calorie constraint, however, accomplishing ketosis could be just as effective.

Together with decreasing the general threat of aging-related illnesses like Alzheimer's and Parkinson's and other persistent illnesses by stabilizing blood sugar level, decreasing cholesterol, and dropping excess weight, ketosis is operating at the cellular level to enhance the body's most important functions by supporting mitochondria.

Mitochondria are the source of power discovered in every cell in the body, and their health is straightly related to your general wellness. In a state of ketosis, mitochondria produce less complimentary radicals and more anti-oxidants. Ketosis can likewise increase the variety of mitochondria in the hippocampus, which might be beneficial to brain function.

In general, the comprehensive advantages of ketosisto make appear to support a healthy body and brain that might extremely well defy aging.

Who should avoid Ketosis?

It's essential not to confuse ketosis with ketoacidosis, which is a deadly problem from type 1 diabetes (and in some cases type 2) that can be triggered from an inadequate quantity of insulin and hazardous concentrations of ketones in the blood. For this reason, you need to speak with a physician prior to trying a keto diet plan if you have type 1 or type 2 diabetes.

You'll likewise wish to look for medical recommendations concerning the security of ketosis if you have any of the lists below conditions:

- Hypertension.
- Liver, kidney, or heart illness.
- History of stomach coronary bypass.
- Pregnant or breastfeeding.
- Any metabolic conditions, like specific enzyme shortages, that can impact how the body produces and utilizes ketones.

How to maintain the state of ketosis.

Ketosis is a procedure that the majority of our bodies can flourish on, and there is a frustrating quantity of research study to support this. Preserving ketosis might be your most tough fight, particularly when you're simply getting begun.

Together with following a constant keto diet plan, you'll wish to make certain you're remaining consuming and hydrating electrolytes. Include periodic fasting, routine workout, exogenous ketones, and MCT oil, along with lots of great sleep, to regularly get the most cognitive and physical advantages out of ketosis-- as you can see there are lots of.

A ketogenic diet is characterized by a metabolic state called "ketosis," in which the body switches life support from carbohydrates to fats. This occurs when there is a deficiency of glucose in the blood when fats are used as fuel. This produces a by-product of metabolism - ketone bodies - soluble organic compounds.

According to studies, ketones are a mobile energy source that slows down aging when a balanced, low-carb, non-refined sugar diet is used. The opposite condition, accelerating aging, occurs when consuming high-calorie "fast food", instant food - "artificial garbage".

Used as an energy source instead of carbohydrates, ketone bodies accumulate in the blood, and when excess concentration is excreted through the urine, this is their advantage. This does not happen when consuming large amounts of glucose, which forms body fat.

Even if the state of ketosis does not occur, ketone bodies are still present in the blood - they are produced in the liver constantly. And when entering ketosis through a diet, the number of ketones increases significantly and the body begins to burn fat instead of glucose. In order not to get confused, you need to understand that ketosis is fundamentally different from ketoacidosis, which threatens life with diabetes.

Types of ketone bodies

There are 3 major types of ketone bodies. To go straight to the point, they are:

Acetoacetate is the main ketone body, an energy-saturated compound produced during normal metabolism. In the process of its oxidation, a large amount of active oxygen is produced - 45 times more than during the oxidation of glucose, and much less "harmful" oxygen. This means that energy supply during ketosis is more powerful, and inflammatory processes are difficult.

Beta-hydroxybutyric acid (3HB, 3-β-hydroxybutyrate, BOMC) is a derivative of acetoacetate formed during its reduction.

In fact, 3HB during the ketone process is reduced to the hydroxyl group, and, in fact, is not a ketone body, but is positioned as such. According to studies, BOMK helps prevent type

2 diabetes due to the ability to be transported into tissues and participate in cell signaling. When bound to surface receptors, BOMK inhibits histone deacetylase, regulates the balance of nicotinic compounds, and regulates the enzymes of the aging process.

"Acetone" - as a ketone body is produced to a lesser extent than the previous types, but this is enough to measure the ketone level in the body. Acetone, being a metabolite of acetoacetate, gives an anticonvulsant effect, and most of it is excreted in the urine.

Production of ketones in the human body

Another very important thing to understand is how the ketones in the body are actually produced. This will help you in making the right decision on how to cater to your body when you are over the age of 50. Our body begins to produce ketones inside the liver cells during a diet with a reduced amount of carbohydrates (up to 20-25 g) and a high-fat content. This occurs through a lipase reaction - the release of fatty acids during hydrolysis, and the transfer of acyl-CoA enzymes through mitochondrial membranes.

Through research, several stages characteristic of the formation of ketones were identified: with lipases, fatty acids in adipose tissue are destroyed; plasma fatty acids are transferred and activated; together with oxidation, fatty acids are transferred to cells.

The other 3 stages are accompanied by the synthesis of ketone bodies:

- Acetoacetyl-CoA is formed.
- Acetoacetate is formed.
- Acetoacetate is restored or destroyed to the "3HB" state.

Otherwise, it looks like this: as soon as a person restricts carbohydrate intake and starts a ketogenic diet, the body is deficient in carbohydrates, begins to search and identifies another source of nutrition for energy production. The best that the body can find is body fat. Adapting to a diet and a transitional period can take up to 2 weeks. During this time, the body, deprived of the intake of new carbohydrates uses the reserves of accumulated glycogen. He will then switch to fat and direct fatty acids into the liver to break them down to ketones for energy.

Benefits of Ketones as energy sources

In addition to the benefits that you may have read in between the sentences of this book, ketones provide additional health benefits:

Fast and stable energy

Ketones directly enter the liver and are quickly processed in it, unlike "slow" glucose traveling through the entire digestive system. That's why when you use fat-containing food, you very quickly - in just a few minutes - "charge your batteries" and you won't wait for hours for an influx of energy.

Much less often, new meals are required, prolonged fasting (for those who practice it) is easier to tolerate when your body has adapted to processing fat and producing ketones. For this reason, during adaptation to fat, "interval starvation" is well perceived by the body.

Such a source of energy makes you slim

Ketones do not form "storage rooms" in the body, unlike glucose. With the excess, excreted in the urine, they are not stored in the form of fat folds on the sides and waist, which by itself ensures harmony for practitioners with such a diet.

The above applies to ketones of exogenous origin (produced not in one's own body, but brought in from an external synthetic source). Ketone supplements included in the ketogenic diet give the body the necessary energy, and the excess is excreted through the urine.

Strengthen and improve brain function

Ketones are also a quick source of fuel for the brain, due to the ability to cross the blood-brain barrier. They also have a beneficial effect on cognitive processes by increasing the number of cellular mitochondria in the brain.

According to a number of studies, ketones are involved in the prevention of Alzheimer's and dementia. They promote energy metabolism and recovery from ischemic stroke by restoring the levels of glutamate and glutamine in the brain due to the carbon they produce.

Normalize blood sugar and regulate weight

Due to ketones, the need for insulin decreases - the glycemic reaction improves because carbohydrates are excluded from consumption. Therefore, there is no spasmodic increase in blood sugar, the risk of diabetes is reduced. The restriction in glucose intake eliminates fat accumulation and excess weight.

Prevent inflammatory processes

The anti-inflammatory effect observed with a ketogenic diet is explained by a decrease in the production of reactive oxygen species (ROS) in ketosis, as well as the lack of glucose in the diet since it is a sugar that often causes inflammation. According to some studies, ketones act as antioxidants, block free radicals, and prevent inflammatory diseases.

Heals the heart

Ketones make up for heart failure by supplementing it with energy - studies conducted in 2016 showed this result. It turns out that fatty acids are necessary for the normalization of cardiac activity.

Ketosis vs ketoacidosis

Although these words are similar, there are significant differences between ketosis and ketoacidosis.

People following a ketogenic diet easily achieve a state of ketosis, it is sometimes called "food ketosis." This condition is generated by the body when carbohydrates are excluded from the diet and replaced with foods with a high proportion of fats, in order to encourage physiology to burn fat as fuel. The consequence of this approach is the destruction of fatty acids, with the formation of a "by-product" of ketones. This condition provides many benefits to human health.

Ketoacidosis is dangerous for people with diabetes - this should not be forgotten. Type 1 diabetics (an autoimmune species) are susceptible to the dangerous and toxic accumulation of ketones, which oxidize the blood and destroy the liver and kidneys. These people depend on skipping insulin injections, and therefore they need to consult a doctor before a keto diet.

Ketone Level Measurement and getting into ketosis

To measure the number of ketones in the blood and respiration, standard ketone counters are used, and for urine.

The main reason for the positive effect of a keto diet is to achieve a state of ketosis. It will be logical to conclude that all women over the age of 50 practicing keto diet, regardless of whether they begin or continue, tend to start the ketosis process as quickly as possible. If you are just starting to take the first steps towards achieving a state of ketosis, you should not rush. Keto - a diet is better to start gradually to give the body to get used to a new state. If you have already practiced ketosis before, but left it because of a vacation, a protracted cheat-mil or drinking alcohol, several proven, effective and **simple** ways can help you return to ketosis.

Ways to return to ketosis

Limit carbohydrates

No matter how trite it may sound, but the first and most important step to achieving ketosis is to limit the intake of pure carbohydrates daily to 20-25 g. This will allow the body to quickly process the glucose supply, and then begin active burning of fats for energy.

Dance

Yes, you heard me right. Dancing at 50 is still achievable. Ketosis can only be achieved by burning glycogen, which is stored in the liver and muscles. Glycogen is the energy reserve of our body, it is his body that burns in the first place, and after that fat is consumed. One of the easiest ways to burn glycogen is to do more cardio workouts. Brisk walking, dancing, running, cycling - all this will have an active effect on glycogen consumption.

Exercise on an empty stomach

Exercising on an empty stomach will enable your body to use the accumulated glycogen and then fat more efficiently since the body will not waste energy on digesting recently taken food. Strength training on large muscle groups (legs, back, shoulders) will be especially useful on an empty stomach, it will increase glycogen consumption even more, which will significantly increase the level of ketones. There is one point - fasting exercises should not be practiced in the first weeks of a low-carb diet.

Intermittent fasting

Fasting will help your body use up glycogen stores faster, because during training you will spend it actively, and there's no more restocking. Be attentive to the general condition of the body, it is worth starving only if you are confident in your own abilities.

Consume enough fat

Eating enough foods that contain saturated fats (olive and coconut oils, avocados, redfish, nuts, etc.), as well as limiting carbohydrate mass in your diet, will help your body quickly adapt to the process of burning fat. Fat will be transformed into ketone bodies to provide energy to the body.

How long does it take to attain ketosis?

The simplest and straight forward answer to this question is that the state of ketosis can be achieved over a period of 3 to 7 days.

Remember that the most important thing on the way to ketosis is the restriction of carbohydrates. If you neglect this rule, the rest will not help you get into ketosis (with the exception of periodic fasting).

KETO FLU: SYMPTOMS, CAUSES AND HOW TO HANDLE IN WOMEN OVER THA AGE OF 50

When choosing a diet over 50 years of age, most people think exclusively about how to lose weight because of the heaviness of the body and increasing the energy level, forgetting about the possible adverse effects. A diet that limits the number of carbohydrates consumed sometimes leads to poor health, provoking the development of a condition called keto-flu. Before changing the diet at 50 years, you need to familiarize yourself with possible side effects.

Keto flu

Keto flu is the body's response to a carbohydrate restriction. Don't be alarmed, this is not a viral disease, although it has similar symptoms. The severity of this condition depends on metabolic flexibility. Most metabolically flexible people have no symptoms of this phenomenon. In others, this condition takes on a pronounced character and requires "therapy".

Keto-diet is based on the mechanism of ketosis when the body uses energy synthesized not from carbohydrates, but from fat reserves.

The slower the transition to a diet that restricts the intake of foods fortified with carbohydrates, the easier the restriction is tolerated.

Keto flu Symptoms

Changes in the food system in women over the age of 50 may provoke the following unpleasant symptoms:

- Headaches and dizziness;
- Physical weakness;
- Body aches;
- Nausea
- Decrease in concentration;
- Loss of motivation;
- Irritability;
- Muscle cramps.

These symptoms are characteristic not only of keto-flu but also colds, so not everyone understands that the reason for this condition is diet.

Causes of keto flu

Keto-flu develops against the background of the use of the body as an energy source of fats, rather than sugars. Switching to a diet with a minimum amount of carbohydrates is fraught with a decrease in insulin levels. Due to this, health improves. This is the goal of the ketogenic diet. With low insulin levels, the liver is mistaken for converting fats into ketones, which the vast majority of cells successfully use instead of sugar. With the active synthesis of energy organisms from ketones and fats, a state of ketosis develops.

The brain and internal organs need time to get used to a new type of fuel. In conditions of lowering insulin levels, more salts and fluids are excreted from the body along with urine. For this reason, in the early days of the ketogenic diet, the urge to use the toilet in a small way is significantly more frequent. This is the basis for the effect of rapid weight loss.

Each person has an individual reaction to a keto diet. Someone feels great, and someone begins to experience unpleasant symptoms, "falling out" of the usual rhythm of life for several days.

The duration of keto-flu depends on how long a person limits himself in carbohydrate intake. If you start "therapy" immediately after the onset of such a condition, improvements will quickly come. The body will soon adapt to changes in nutrition. In advanced cases, the condition may worsen a recovery may take several weeks.

How to treat keto flu

There are several ways to "treat" keto-flu. They come down to recommendations, compliance with which can improve the condition.

The tips are as follows:

- Drink more fluids.

- Include electrolytes in the diet.

- Eat more fats.

- Get enough sleep.

- Gently exercise and meditate.

- Take activated charcoal and an exogenous ketone supplement.

Water is the best helper in the fight against keto-flu. Before drinking liquid, it is recommended to stir a small amount of unrefined salt in it. When determining the optimal amount of daily water intake, it is necessary to be guided by body weight. The physiological norm per 1 kilogram is 30 ml. To maintain water balance per day, you need to drink about 1.5-2 liters of liquid.

It is recommended that bone broth be included in the diet, following a diet that limits the intake of carbohydrate-rich foods. From this dish, the body will receive a serving of fluid and electrolytes - sodium and potassium. This will eliminate the discomfort experienced at the cellular level.

Replenishing electrolytes is a great way to feel better. Magnesium, sodium, and potassium can be consumed as additives. They are also found in many products. Potassium is rich in fish, leafy greens. Magnesium spinach, chicken and beef. This component is effective for symptoms of keto-flu, such as muscle cramps, dizziness, and a feeling of tiredness.

MCT oil is the main supplier of healthy fats, it must also be present in the diet. Increasing the amount of fat consumed speeds up the period of addiction - the body will burn fat faster than sugar.

A good night's sleep will help defeat keto-flu. It provides control over the level of cortisol, due to this, negative symptoms are reduced. You need to sleep at least 7-9 hours a day.

Soft workouts also help reduce cortisol levels. They are especially effective at the initial stage of the diet. It is recommended to do yoga, take leisurely walks. Adapting to a keto diet accelerates meditation.

To cleanse the body of toxins using activated carbon. This drug not only stimulates the elimination of toxic substances but also improves the general condition.

In the fight against fatigue that occurs in many who go on a keto diet, exogenous ketone supplements help. They give a boost of energy, increase the concentration of ketones in the blood. Such supplements are recommended to be taken in the first 3-5 days of symptoms of keto-flu. The main thing is not to overdo it with dosages and remember that they are not able to replace a full ketone diet.

If these tips do not help, it is worth slightly increasing the number of carbohydrates consumed.

The transition to a keto diet should be smooth - this will prevent the development of side effects from limiting carbohydrates. The condition characteristic of keto-flu can be dealt with if you follow simple recommendations.

BENEFITS OF KETO DIET YOU DIDN'T KNOW ABOUT

Over the past ten years, hundreds of studies have been carried out that confirm the same data: the intake of healthy fats is not harmful to health and, conversely, is more beneficial than a high-carb diet. So let's talk with you about the benefits of keto.

Consuming any kind of carbohydrate raises blood sugar. The spike may occur faster or slower depending on the type of carbohydrate (based on the glycemic index), but the spike will happen anyway.

Bursts of blood sugar cause strong insulin bursts to control bursts. Continuous insulin releases lead to fat accumulation and insulin resistance. After many years, this cycle can lead to prediabetes, metabolic syndrome, and even type 2 diabetes.

We are beginning to realize that carbohydrates in large quantities are much more harmful than previously thought, while most fats are good for health.

The nutritional picture is changing. Low-carb and similar dietary groups are growing, and the revolution in nutrition is beginning. We are becoming aware of the harmful effects of our close relationship with excess sugar and carbohydrates.

Other Benefits

Long-term benefits

Studies have consistently shown that those who follow a low-carb, high-fat diet, rather than the opposite, are high-carb and low-fat diets:

Lose more weight and fat.

Have healthy levels of beneficial cholesterol (HDL and high LDL)

Reduce your blood sugar and insulin resistance (often reversing prediabetes and type 2 diabetes)

Experience a decrease in appetite

Notice a decrease in triglycerides (blood fat molecules that cause heart disease)

A significant decrease in blood pressure is observed, which leads to a decrease in the risk of cardiovascular disease and stroke

Following low-carb or ketogenic diets helps you lose more weight than any low-fat diet.

Short-term benefits

Keto diet benefits not only in the long run! When you eat keto, you can expect:

Loss of subcutaneous and visceral fat;

Stable energies throughout the day;

A long feeling of satiety after eating, fewer snacks and overeating.

A prolonged feeling of satiety and constant flashes of energy are the results of the fact that most calories come from fat, which is more slowly digested and more caloric.

Eating low-carb foods also eliminates blood glucose surges. You will no longer have sudden drops in blood sugar that make you feel weak and disoriented.

I perfectly understand that a person is not afraid to die until he begins to die. And we live in complete confidence in our immortality, but still, I want to touch on the topic of diseases in which a ketogenic nutrition system can help you.

The worst diseases of the 21st century are cardiovascular and cancer.

If you play associations now, what associations can lead to the word "cardiovascular disease"? Death, obesity, overweight, stroke, heart attack, coronary heart disease, heart failure, arrhythmia, diabetes ... the list will be very long. And we understand that 99.5 out of 100 people will fall into this risk zone.?

To date, it has been proven that 4 factors lead to the development of the worst diseases, especially in women over 50 years: oxidation, inflammation, sugar, and stress. And they are all interconnected. By eliminating one of the factors, we can weaken, or completely eliminate, the influence of the other. Keto definitely removes the influence of the factor-sugar.

In order to remove the other 3, keto should be combined with a rejection of gluten, with combination therapy to maintain intestinal health, and therapy to reduce the risk of oxidative stress.

Yes, all this is not easy, but let's eat an elephant piece by piece.

WHAT HAPPENS TO THE BODY DURING KETO DIET

During a keto-diet, the following occurs with the body:

With the minimal intake of carbohydrates and, consequently, glucose, the liver begins to process existing fats into ketones, providing a person with a gradual and gentle process of losing weight.

Switching the body to burning fat instead of using carbohydrates provokes a condition reminiscent of the symptoms of flu or a cold (dizziness, nausea, muscle discomfort, headache, sleep disturbance, etc.). In about a week, these symptoms will disappear and the body will fully adapt to the new nutrition system.

Further, in the process of losing weight, cravings for sweets and appetite as a whole decrease, sleep quality improves, energy levels increase, and a person begins to actively get rid of accumulated body fat.

Thanks to ketosis, losing weight does not feel hunger and is saturated with those portions of food (mainly proteins and fats) that are consumed during the day.

Fat folds begin to dissolve a little and the relief of the muscles are drawn (especially when playing sports). The body becomes fit and slim.

All these factors together contribute to weight loss.

BENEFITS OF A KETO DIET

The keto diet has the following advantages:

Losing excess weight in a relatively short time. Moreover, excess weight after refusing this power system does not return, reliably securing itself at the reached mark.

A constant feeling of satiety. Since the basis of the ketogenic nutrition system is high-calorie foods (low-fat varieties of fish and meat, milk and dairy products, vegetables), the body is quickly saturated and the person does not think about food.

Serves as the prevention of diabetes. Dietary foods help lower blood sugar.

Suitable for people with epilepsy. Such a nutrition program helps to reduce the frequency of seizures in the disease, therefore, it is recommended as an epileptic drug as therapeutic nutrition.

It has a positive effect on blood pressure and cholesterol. Hypertensive patients note normalization of pressure and overall well-being (due to a decrease in "bad" cholesterol in the blood).

Increases brain activity. Ketones produced by the liver increase the energy level in the body and improve concentration.

Improves the condition of the skin, giving it a radiant and well-groomed appearance.

Keto-diet is an effective nutritional system, which implies the rejection of carbohydrates and daily intake of protein and fatty foods. As a result, the body begins to actively burn accumulated body fat and a person loses weight. But before starting a diet, it is recommended to consult a therapist and undergo an examination to make sure there are no contraindications.

KETO EGGS FASTING FOR WOMEN OVER 50

An egg fast on a keto diet is a short-term period lasting no more than 5 days. It is designed to overcome the state of the plateau, which is characterized by stopping the decrease in body weight and freezing it on one bar in women over 50. Its reduction does not occur, despite the exact adherence to a selected diet and the performance of daily activity in older women. Using an egg diet, you can help the body accelerate metabolic processes and get rid of excess body fat in problem areas.

Rules

Egg fasting includes eating eggs, fat, and cheese. The short-term diet is based on the use of a small amount of protein and carbohydrates. As a result, a state of ketosis occurs.

The cells of the body do not get enough carbohydrates, and to compensate for the lack of energy, the process of splitting your own fat occurs. The liver converts fat into ketone bodies and fatty acids, which replace glucose in the body.

The daily egg diet includes:

6-12 eggs. The amount depends on age and build.

• 1 tbsp. of fat per egg. You can use; butter, coconut, homemade mayonnaise or lard.

• 200 g of cheese per day or 30 g for each egg.

From a liquid drink:

• Water

- Tea

- Coffee

With an egg diet, vitamin C is absent in food. It is replaced with a slice of lemon added to tea or plain water.

Basic rules for consuming foods during fasting:

- The first egg should be eaten within half an hour after morning awakening.
- Alternate meals every 3-5 hours.
- Do not eat 3 hours before bedtime.
- Eat at least 6 eggs per day.

The obligatory rule is to strictly follow the nutrition plan and is even in the case when there is no appetite and there is a feeling of satiety.

The benefit of keto egg fasting

An egg is a product rich in composition. It contains all the necessary substances for the full functioning of the body. During the diet, there is no harm to the body due to a lack of nutrients.

Egg fasting does not cause a feeling of hunger and stress, which often accompanies it.

Benefits for the body with a short-term egg diet:

• Fat deposits in problem areas go away.

• There is a habit of eating in small portions. It is fixed and after the end of egg fasting, there is moderate consumption of food throughout the day.

• The body starts metabolic processes that do not end at the end of the diet.

• Slimming does not deplete muscle fibers.

Egg fasting is superior in its effectiveness to a diet based on lower calorie intake from the daily allowance.

In order for the processes running in the body not to sleep, but to continue to burn fats effectively, you need to switch to proper nutrition after fasting and observe the keto diet. In this system, you can't eat or need to limit: sugar, bread, pasta, cereals, sweet fruits, and vegetables. But be sure to eat a large amount of fat and cheese of any kind.

Downsides of keto egg fasting

Egg fasting is safe for healthy people. The only negative, for 5 days you can get tired of constantly eating eggs.

You cannot use the diet:
• During pregnancy and breastfeeding.

- The presence of any gastrointestinal disease.

- Diabetes mellitus type 1 and 2.

- Diseases of the gallbladder and bile ducts.

- High blood cholesterol.

- Depressive conditions.

- The period of increased emotional and physical stress.

During fasting, constipation can occur. For its prevention, it is worth consuming more than 1.5 liters of fluid per day.

Egg fasting recipes

In order to diversify the use of the same products, you need to alternate them. The daily diet includes 3 meals: breakfast, lunch, and dinner, as well as two snacks between them. As a snack, cheese of any kind is used. It can be grated, cut into strips or cut into cubes and strung on a skewer.

Each menu consists of the following components:

1st day:

• Use the eggs to cook an omelet with butter.

• Hardboiled eggs.

• Pancakes made from eggs with wheat flour and butter.

2nd day:

• Pancake based on eggs and cheese, fried in butter.

• Egg salad flavored with homemade mayonnaise.

• Baked bun. It is worth cutting the crust. if it formed at the bottom.

3rd day:

• Fry eggs with butter.

• Be limited to cheese.

• Hardboiled eggs.

4th day:

• Omelet.

• Hardboiled eggs.

• Wafer sticks prepared in a special kitchen appliance.

5th day:

• Omelet.

• Salad seasoned with mayonnaise.

• Cheese casserole.

Morning meals are combined with black tea or coffee. It is allowed to drink a small number of carbonated drinks during the day.

By observing an egg fast based on a keto diet, you can lose a few pounds in a short period of time, start metabolic processes and at the same time not experience a strong feeling of hunger, and hence stress. During this period, the body starts the mechanism of burning its own reserves of fat in the most problematic places. These include the stomach, buttocks, and hips. Here, the excess volume will gradually decrease.

BENEFITS OF KETO DIET FOR WOMEN OVER 50

The goal of the ketogenic diet is to "get into ketosis". Ketosis, as mentioned, is a metabolic state in which your body runs out of glycogen (practically sugar) and instead uses primarily fatty acids for energy.

In response to this change, your liver produces ketone bodies that provide your body and brain with clean and sustainable energy.

To achieve this goal, you must adhere to a strict low / no-carb, moderate protein, and high-fat diet. It requires a certain degree of discipline and a special keto diet plan that you can orient yourself towards.

With this brief summary, we can now take a closer look at the list of benefits of ketosis and low-carb.

While many other diets have only one benefit (which would ideally be weight loss), the ketogenic diet offers a variety of benefits for your physical and mental performance and health.

The reason for this is the fact that the energy generation from fatty acids and ketone bodies is significantly more effective than the combustion of glycogen or carbohydrates.

First of all the most important advantages and positive effects of a low-carb diet or the ketogenic diet:

- Lose weight faster and increase fat burning
- Improved sleep quality and better regeneration

- More mitochondria and improved mitochondrial performance
- Lower insulin and blood sugar levels

Here is the complete list of the best-known benefits of ketogenic nutrition, including scientific studies and explanations:

Accelerated fat burning

Refraining from sugar carbohydrates is one of the most effective ways to lose as much fat as possible and thus excess body weight in a short time.

The reason for this is that low-carb diets drain excess water from your body in the first step, then lower your insulin level and ultimately reduce your hunger/appetite.

Ketosis then figuratively transforms your body into a fat-burning machine that is active 24 hours a day, 7 days a week in women over 50 years.

Stable and low blood sugar level

Millions of women over 50 years worldwide suffer from diabetes or high insulin resistance. The good news for these people is that the ketogenic diet can offer them some benefits.

Avoiding carbohydrates can dramatically reduce your blood sugar level and thus prevent tiredness or hunger attacks as well as diabetes in women over 50 years of age.

Increased endurance

At this old age, endurance can increase their performance through ketosis. This is due to the fact that energy generation from ketones and fatty acids requires less oxygen and is generally more efficient.

Better sleep quality

Sleep and especially deep sleep have been proven to be one of the most important processes in our body. Here too, ketosis can work wonders! When you start the ketogenic diet you will notice that you got out of bed faster and more relaxed in the morning. This is primarily due to the fact that ketosis, on the one hand, activates the cell's internal "garbage disposal" and on the other hand leads to efficient energy generation.

Improved brain functions

Another well-researched benefit of ketogenic nutrition is the enhancement of brain functions such as memory, concentration, or focus. The older you grow, the less brain function you are likely to have. If you are on an average diet that is not specifically suited for your age, then you may experience brain deterioration. There are a number of human studies that have confirmed the positive effects of ketosis on the memory of adults. In addition, ketosis leads to increased production of mitochondria in the human brain, which can increase the concentration of ATP in your brain, and especially in your hippocampus.

Higher basal metabolic rate and energy consumption

Your basal metabolic rate in the amount of energy your body needs each day to keep the most important functions in your body running. Women over the age of 50 usually struggle to achieve basal metabolic rates. There are some studies that have linked low carb or ketogenic diets to higher metabolic rates. This means that you can lose weight faster in the long term or define your body or muscles.

Nutritious diet

Foods you should eat on the ketogenic diet include fish, vegetables, high-quality meat, and other unprocessed foods. These foods are fundamentally rich in minerals and important nutrients that contribute to the health and performance of your body.

Lower blood pressure

Equally exciting: hypertension patients can benefit from a ketogenic diet.
researchers have confirmed that a low-carb diet and forms of the ketogenic diet can reduce some important risk factors for various heart diseases. This also includes lower blood pressure.

Stronger mitochondria

Mitochondria are the cellular power plants of our bodies. Without it, we would run out of energy within a few minutes. Much of our health, performance and immune system depends on the function of our mitochondria.

Slower aging process

One way to slow our body's aging is to reduce oxidative stress. Interestingly, a low insulin level leads to less oxidative stress. Refraining from sugar and other carbohydrates as part of a ketogenic diet will lower your blood sugar and insulin levels sustainably. which in turn will measurably and noticeably slow down your aging process.

Faster and stronger satiety

Many diets do one thing above all: a constant feeling of hunger. The ketogenic diet is different here - because it has been proven that it can lead to a stronger feeling of satiety, which also occurs even faster.

Several studies annually prove that the absence of carbohydrates and the consumption of more fat and protein leads to less hunger and fewer calories.

This allows you to burn more fat in less time - without the uncomfortable feeling of constant and pervasive hunger!

Fasting becomes much easier

Each of us knows the feeling when we forego our lunch or simply forget an evening meal because of all the work.

With a normal diet, most people find it difficult to do without any form of food for 12 hours - even though fasting can have an unbelievable number of health benefits. It is different in ketosis: it is no longer a problem if you have to do without food for 12, 16 or even 24 hours. This will make sustained or intermittent fasting (16-hour daily fasting) much easier for you.

Better mood & mood

Google's search for "Autism + Ketosis" leads us to hundreds of blog posts and personal testimonials, all of which talk about the positive effects of the ketogenic diet on people with autism. This effect is caused, among other things, by the increased formation of GABA and serotonin in the course of ketosis. The release of these happiness hormones, in turn, means that keto dieters often report an improved mood. GABA (gamma-aminobutyric acid) is a naturally occurring amino acid that acts as a neurotransmitter in the human brain. Neurotransmitters are the messenger substances in our body that transmit signals of all kinds from nerve cells to nerve cells. Serotonin is a neurotransmitter (messenger) that is produced in your nerve cells. It ensures smooth signal transmission between your nerve cells. Serotonin is found primarily in the human digestive tract, although smaller amounts can also be detected in the blood platelets and within the entire nervous system. It is the result of the biochemical conversion of the amino acid L-tryptophan. A protein building block (L-tryptophan) is combined with another chemical reactor, creating 5-hydroxytryptamine (5-HT). GABA acts as a so-called inhibitory neurotransmitter because it blocks or slows down the transmission of certain signals.

Another convincing reason to avoid sugar and simple carbohydrates in the future!

Faster weight loss

It has been scientifically proven that low-carb and high-fat diets are THE most effective way to lose a lot of weight and fat deposits in a short amount of time. On the one hand, this has to do with the fact that excess water (which is bound to carbohydrates and glycogen) is excreted.

On the other hand, you are turning your body into an efficient fat-burning machine. In this way, you will burn fat faster and more effectively in the long term and lose weight.

Higher HDL cholesterol

HDL cholesterol (high-density lipoprotein) is often referred to as good cholesterol. The higher the amount of HDL, relative to the "bad" LDL, the lower the risk of heart disease. Due to the high consumption of healthy fatty acids in the course of the ketogenic diet, you can increase the amount of "good" HDL cholesterol and thus prevent heart diseases.

Increased libido

Ketosis can significantly increase the quality of life for men through increased testosterone levels and more libido. This effect becomes stronger the more high-quality fats (MCT, coconut fat, etc.) you consume as a man in ketosis. A good argument to buy a high-quality MCT oil as quickly as possible!

Lower insulin levels

Low-carb diets and the ketogenic diet are particularly beneficial for people with diabetes and insulin resistance - these complaints affect several million people worldwide. Studies have shown that people with diabetes can reduce their insulin levels by up to 50 percent with a low / no-carb diet.

Get up faster in the morning

Because of the improved quality of sleep we wrote about at the beginning of the book, many ketogenic dieters report more energy and willpower to get out of bed in the morning. In many experiences, this is one of the first positive effects that you will notice at the beginning of the ketogenic diet.

Improved LDL cholesterol levels

People with too high an LDL level are more likely to have a heart attack in the course of their lives. In ketosis, the average size of the LDL particles increases, while the absolute number of particles decreases. The larger the LDL particles, the lower the risk of a heart attack. Accordingly, by avoiding sugar and carbohydrates, you can reduce the risk of a heart attack!

Reduces symptoms of allergies

Allergies are one of the common day-to-day challenges of women over 50 years face. Ketosis balances and calms the human immune system. Since an allergy is nothing more than an overreaction of the immune system, ketosis can reduce the symptoms of allergies.

Ketosis has an anti-catabolic effect

Athletes, in particular, are afraid of losing hard-earned muscle mass in ketosis - don't worry, this is not the case if you consume the right keto foods! Ketones have an anti-catabolic effect in your body. This means that they signal your body that it should lose fat, not muscles. This makes as much sense from an evolutionary perspective. Because in times of food shortage, our ancestors needed their muscles to be able to go hunting again.

MEASURING KETOSIS

You naturally desire to know whether you are currently in ketosis or not and whether the benefits of ketosis have currently begun when you start eating keto or the ketogenic way. In addition to the typical indications of ketosis, there are numerous methods to properly determine the variety of ketone bodies in your metabolic process.

The 3 major methods to determine ketosis are:

- Urine measuring strips for determining the ketone bodies in your urine

- Measuring the ketone bodies in your blood

- Measuring the ketone bodies in your breath

In the course of this book, we will present you to these 3 measurement methods in more information, explain in detail how they work and support you in choosing the optimum variation.

Strips of urine approach

Urine strips are the most convenient and least expensive method to measure ketosis. For beginners, this version also offers the essential accuracy to identify the proper stage of ketosis with a reasonably high possibility.

There is no point in doing complicated blood tests if you have just begun ketogenic nutrition. If you want to understand the nuances of ketosis at an innovative stage, these tests only become intriguing.

Urine strips are exceptionally easy to use. You hold the strips in your urine for a few seconds and after 15 to 20 seconds the color of the determining fields changes depending on the variety of ketone bodies in your urine.

The color of the urine strips usually turns redder as the variety of ketone bodies in your urine boosts. A light pink shows a low production of ketone bodies. A deep dark red suggests that you are well advanced in ketosis.

Urine strips are an excellent method to figure out whether you remain in ketosis or not, however, they lack the precision to accurately figure out the number of ketone bodies in your blood in the mmol range.

Instead, they determine the level of acetoacetate in your urine. This type of ketone body is not fully used by your body for energy, however, it is excreted in the urine. The residues can be identified here using appropriate techniques.

The longer you are in ketosis, the more effectively your body can use ketone bodies in your organism and the less precise this method of determining ketosis ends up being.

If you are entirely in ketosis for the very first time, the urine strip is most likely to turn dark red in the first test. After a few weeks, despite high ketone levels in your blood, you will only see a light pink color with urine strips.

While lots of people think this is a bad indication, this development suggests that your body can metabolize the ketone bodies in your organism more effectively. For that reason, urine strips are a relatively imprecise technique to determine your ketone worths objectively, specifically in the long term.

The main advantages of urine strips are that they are easy to use and economical to buy. You can order them straight from Amazon for a few euros and utilize them without much prior knowledge.

The main downside is their mistake. On the one hand, the results become a growing number of incorrect the longer you remain in ketosis and on the other hand the level of your hydration can cause different measurement results with the exact same development of ketosis.

Blood test method

Determining gadgets that determine the development of ketosis straight based on the number of ketone bodies in your blood is, in contrast to urine strips, far more accurate. They show a specific real-time value of the ketone bodies in your blood. They are also used in the kept track of and reliable clinical research studies.

Their disadvantage is the high cost of the device itself and the running costs of the individual test strips. While the purchase price of the device changes over time to the number of measurements, the cost of 1 euro per test strip remains the same. However, if you want to expect accurate results, you have to be willing to invest this amount. Another small disadvantage is the different measurement accuracy of the blood tests in relation to different devices and test strips. The number of ketone values that the measuring devices produce varies enormously depending on the device and test strips - even if they were produced by the same manufacturer.

In addition, you must note that you have to give yourself a small prick in your index finger for each measurement. Even though most people can overlook this little pain, you should be aware of it.

You can regularly find good deals online for cheap measuring devices. However, the manufacturers build their devices in such a way that they can usually only be operated with the brand's own measuring strips - which in turn can really cost money in the long term. So make a smart decision and include the price per test strip in your bill before buying the device.

Breath tests

Devices with which you can measure ketosis through the air you breathe have become increasingly popular in recent years - and not just because of their simplicity. You simply connect the device to your computer via USB. Then you blow hard into the device. As a result, the system measures the acetate content in your breathing air. This gives you a pretty good idea of how many ketone bodies you have in your bloodstream. These breath tests usually cost between 120 and 170 euros, making them the most expensive option for measuring ketone bodies. If you're on the ketogenic diet, i recommend that you wait until you get to a more advanced stage. Then it makes sense to invest the above amount in a higher accuracy of the measurements. Then when you are at a point where you have to choose between a blood meter and a breath meter, I would advise you to pay the higher amount in advance, instead of having to pay money for individual test strips again and again, as in the case of blood meters, In the course of the scientific application of the breath meters, a relatively stable correlation between the amount of acetate in your breath and the number of ketone bodies in your blood has emerged. Even though breath tests are much more accurate than urine tests, they show a larger spread compared to direct blood tests. This can lead to inaccurate results and incorrect conclusions about the stage of ketosis. If lower long-term costs are more important to you than the last 5 percent accuracy, you should choose a breath test. If you only value the highest possible measuring accuracy, it makes sense to invest more money in a blood measuring device and enough measuring strips.

BEST KETO ZONE FOR WOMEN OVER 50

There are several stages of ketosis that are solely defined by the number of ketone bodies in your bloodstream. Basically, you can say that more ketone bodies in your blood also indicate faster weight loss and better mental performance.

Since blood tests have the highest accuracy of all measurement variants, we will use them as a primary example. If you can have less than 0.75 mmol of ketone bodies per liter of blood, you are basically not in ketosis.

Above 0.75 mmol / L one speaks of ketosis. In this area, you can also feel the classic symptoms of keto flu during the first few days.

You can use the following graphic and the measurements of your breath or blood tests to measure whether you are on the way to ketosis or not. Often the process of ketosis takes longer than expected and you have to try a few things from exercise to the right foods and other factors to get into ketosis in the long term and stay in ketosis.

If you're already deep in ketosis, you should be more careful. Values above 3.0 mmol / L indicate that your body produces a large number of ketone bodies. However, the positive effects on your body and mind are the same as the values of 2.5 mmol / L.

If you regularly measure values above 3.0 mmol / L, this may indicate that you are consuming too few calories from your diet. Ketosis can also occur when people are hungry and generally consume too few calories. This is not the point and you should replace missing calories with high-quality fats or protein.

Ultimately, as a kind of marginal note, we should also talk about high ketone values, Values above 6.0 mmol / L usually indicate a dangerous metabolic state called ketoacidosis. Even if it is almost impossible to reach such a high level as part of a standard ketogenic diet, you should measure the stage of ketosis regularly and in the event of increased ketone levels, consult a doctor immediately!

MAJOR FOODS FOR KETO DIET AT 50

The ketogenic diet limits the carbohydrate intake, depending on age, gender and weight, to 20-50 grams per day. At first glance, this can be a little intimidating, but if you become familiar with ketogenic-friendly foods, it will automatically work much better.

I have put together an ultimate list for you that you can always use. These healthy foods are gold pieces in your ketogenic diet. Healthy, tasty and still low in carbohydrates - perfect!

Meat and poultry

Meat and poultry should be your go-to staples on a ketogenic diet. Fresh meat and poultry do not contain any carbohydrates, but a lot of vitamin B and important minerals such as potassium, selenium, and zinc.

Meat and poultry also provide an excellent source of high-quality protein. Protein not only keeps you full with a low-carbohydrate diet but also helps to maintain your existing muscle mass, especially when losing weight.

Ideally, you only try to eat the meat of animals that feed on fresh grass. Because their meat contains a lot of the healthy omega-3 fatty acids, antioxidants, and conjugated linoleic acid. These, in turn, help to reduce body fat and body weight and sometimes have anti-inflammatory effects.

Avocados

Avocados contain one of the healthiest fats because they are rich in unsaturated fatty acids. These can be used as long-term energy sources and, thanks to their high fiber content, also fill you up for a long time. Due to the many fibers, the regular consumption of avocados also affects regulated digestion.

The power fruit is a real miracle cure and also helps to replenish the body's electrolyte storage. This is especially important for athletes and athletes who lose a lot of electrolytes due to constant sweating after a sports session.

150 grams of the fruit contains 975 milligrams of potassium, a mineral that regulates the body's fluid balance. This is super important if you are on a ketogenic diet, as the body only gets a few carbohydrates.

With a low-carb diet, the body stores less water and electrolytes, which can lead to a lack of fluids, dizziness, poor circulation and other symptoms of keto flu.

Nuts and seeds

As a rule, nuts and seeds all contain a lot of healthy fatty acids. Each nut and each seed naturally bring different nutrients with it.

For example, a handful of almonds already covers 10 percent of your daily calcium requirements, while the same amount of pumpkin seeds covers more than a quarter of your daily zinc requirements.

Top tip: grab a few raw vegetable sticks and enjoy them with a few spoons of peanut or almond butter. A healthy snack with high-fat content is the perfect snack for a ketogenic diet! Check out the list of the carbohydrate content of the major nuts and seeds at a glance (28 grams per serving):

- Almonds: 6 grams
- Brazil nut : 3 grams
- Cashew nuts: 9 grams

- Macadamia nut: 4 grams

- Pecans: 4 grams

- Pistachio nuts: 8 grams

- Walnuts: 4 grams

- Chia seeds: 12 grams

- Flax seeds: 8 grams

- Pumpkin seeds: 5 grams

- Sesame seeds: 7 grams

Dark chocolate and cocoa powder

Chocolate at 50? Yes, you heard me right! Good news for chocolate lovers: chocolate can also be part of a ketogenic diet! This specifically applies to women over the age of 50 years. It is important, however, that only dark chocolate with a cocoa content of at least 70% is chosen.

For example, 28 grams of 100% cocoa chocolate has only 3 grams of carbohydrates. The same amount of chocolate with 70-85%

cocoa contains up to 10 grams of carbohydrates.

The cardiovascular system

Drinking dark chocolate in moderation can help improve cardiovascular health in women over 50, scientists say. A group of scientists led by David Grassi at the University of Aquila, Italy, conducted a randomized clinical trial to compare the effects of dark chocolate with white on blood pressure and glucose and insulin absorption. The study involved a group of 15 people with a typical Italian diet, and they received 100 grams of dark chocolate per day, which contains about 500 milligrams of polyphenols, for 15 days, or as much white chocolate, presumably not containing polyphenols.

Researchers found that dark chocolate is responsible for lowering blood pressure and improving insulin sensitivity in study participants. This data, published in the March 2005 edition of the American Journal of Clinical Nutrition, was a prerequisite for the results of other studies evaluating the health benefits of other polyphenolic products, such as green tea.

Plaque protection in women over the age of 50

An animal study was conducted at Otak University in Japan and found that portions of cocoa beans, the main ingredient in dark chocolate, kill bacteria in the mouth and protect against plaque and caries. The results of this study are a guide published more than ten years ago, which were carried out with the support of several other studies. Researchers reported that rinsing the mouth with a decoction of cocoa beans was an effective way to reduce plaque in children. Cocoa appears to attack plaque by inhibiting an enzyme that plays a key role in plaque formation. Don't forget that at the age of 50 years upwards, plaque is a common disease.

Natural cough eradication in women over the age of 50

Since women who are 50 years and above have a low immune defense system, they need a painless and healthy solution. In 2004, Professor Peter Barnes and his colleagues at Imperial College London conducted a study showing cocoa to be more effective in fighting persistent coughs than medications. Ten volunteers who participated in this British study were divided into three groups. The first group was given tablets containing theobromine, a cocoa derivative, the second group received traditional cough suppressants containing codeine, and the third group was given a placebo. After taking the drugs, the participants inhaled gas containing capsaicin, a component of chili pepper, which, as you know, causes a cough. Those who received theobromine had a lower cough level. Moreover, cocoa derivatives have fewer side effects than conventional cough medicines.

Dark chocolate is a powerful source of minerals for women over the age of 50

This chocolate variety also enriches the body with a range of minerals, including iron, magnesium, zinc, selenium, copper, phosphorus, potassium and manganese. Minerals act both individually and synergistically, performing hundreds of tasks in the human body. They help provide, for example, protection of nerves, bones, arteries, hair, nails, skin and the immune system.

100g of dark chocolate with 70-85% cocoa contains:

11 g fiber

67% of the recommended daily intake of iron

58% of the recommended daily intake of magnesium

98% of the suggested day-to-day consumption of magnesium

A big quantity of zinc, phosphorus, and selenium

All these nutrients come with 600 calories, for this factor dark chocolate, like the other, is much better to consume in small amounts.

A German research study performed on 24 ladies between the ages of 18 and 65 revealed that ladies who got chocolate flavonoids had 15 percent less inflammation from UV direct exposure after 6 weeks and 25 percent after 12 weeks of consuming chocolate. The advantage for ladies is indisputable of this fantastic dark chocolate, to their fantastic enjoyment.

Tiredness and exhaustion

Females over the age of 50 are regularly experiencing tiredness and fatigue. A research study performed by a group of scientists led by Professor Stephen Atkin of Hull York Medical School concluded that the research study individuals were less tired after consuming dark chocolate (85 percent cocoa) daily for 8 weeks, however, started to feel worn out once again when were transformed to cocoa-free food. Sleep disruption is a typical condition amongst individuals with fatigue syndrome and one possible description for the research study results is that dark chocolate can enhance sleep amongst research study individuals because of its capability to increase brain levels of serotonin, a neurotransmitter that controls sleep and state of mind.

Dark chocolate advantages for weight-loss for females

If they consumed chocolate every day, a group of German scientists discovered that individuals on a low-carb diet plan lost 10 percent much faster. Dark chocolate can aid with weight reduction, supporting blood glucose levels by managing cravings and decreasing food yearnings. Dark chocolate flavonoids help in reducing insulin resistance and avoid blood sugar level spikes, avoiding overindulging.

Research Studies at Queen Margaret University have actually revealed motivating outcomes on how dark chocolate impacts the metabolic process of carbs and fats. Dark chocolate has a remarkable impact on how the body manufactures fats, consequently decreasing the absorption of carbs and fats, triggering a sensation of fullness.

To take pleasure in the health advantages of consuming bitter chocolate, you must attempt this tasty healthy dish consisting of chili peppers. For optimum advantages, choose soy milk instead of cow milk, as there is proof that dairy items minimize a few of the advantageous results of cocoa.

Ingredients:

- 2 cups of soy milk (optional).

- 2 teaspoons walking stick sugar.

- 1/2 tablespoon vanilla.

- 1 little red chili split longitudinally and eliminate the seeds.

- 1 cinnamon stick.

- 40 grams of dark chocolate, grated.

Preparation:

In a little pan, mix warm milk with sugar, vanilla, cinnamon, and chili peppers prior to steaming. Beat with grated chocolate and continue to boil till the chocolate has actually melted. Eliminate the vanilla and pepper pods.

Fish.

Fish and seafood are additional repaired points of a ketogenic diet plan. A great deal of fat, couple of carbs and a high material of vitamin B, selenium and potassium - fish types, such as. the salmon, are for that reason perfect for the ketogenic diet plan.

Since the various fruits have various carbs, with seafood you have to be mindful. Shrimp and other crab animals consist of. practically no carbs, clams or mussels for it once again.

Seafood is absolutely ideal for the ketogenic diet plan, however, you need to pick it thoroughly to keep carbs low.

Here is a summary of the carbohydrate material in one serving (100 grams) of popular seafood:

- Clams: 5 grams.

- Oysters: 4 grams.

- Mussels: 7 grams.

- Octopus: 4 grams.

- Squid: 3 grams.

Preferably, you attempt to eat at least 2 portions of seafood a week!

Eggs.

We have actually gone over eggs and their advantages, however simply a little wrap-up. Eggs are cheap, simple to prepare and can be prepared in several methods. Eggs are not just scrumptious, they likewise bring plenty of crucial nutrients such as choline with them.

The egg yolk supplies a perfect source of choline, a compound that has cell protective functions. Choline likewise plays a significant function in enhancing the brain, state of mind, metabolic process and memory, according to the National Health Institute (NIH).

Eggs are likewise among the few foods that have a high vitamin D material, hence considerably supporting eye and bone functions and keeping cholesterol levels low.

Cheese.

There are numerous kinds of various cheeses - and thank God all of them have low carbs and a great deal of fat, making them the ideal buddy in ketosis.

A serving of cheddar cheese (around 28 grams) includes just 1 gram of carbs, 7 grams of fat and 20% of the advised everyday calcium requirement.

Cheese has a somewhat greater portion of saturated fatty acids, however, research studies reveal that this does not position an increased danger of cardiovascular disease. Some research studies even reveal that routine cheese usage even safeguards versus heart problem.

Cheese likewise includes conjugated linoleic acid (CLA), a fat that promotes weight loss and prefers a specified body.

Low carbohydrate veggies & fruits.

Fruits and veggies are an important part of a ketogenic diet plan. With a ketogenic diet plan, nevertheless, you ought to pick the veggies thoroughly, as numerous likewise have a remarkably high carb material.

There is nobody ideal, principle. If you pick the veggies with care, you can quickly consist of most ranges in your ketogenic diet plan.

You need to restrict the following foods:

Veggies with a high carb material. Onions, parsnips, garlic, mushrooms, and pumpkin are consisted of.

Nightshade household. These consist of eggplants, peppers, and tomatoes.

Citrus fruits, consisting of limes, limes, and orange juice or peel in water.

Attempt to prevent starchy veggies and fruits such as potatoes or bananas totally.

In general, whatever that grows under the ground has more carbs and ought to be restricted in the ketogenic diet plan.

Olive oil.

Olive oil includes fat that is abundant in monounsaturated fats and oleic acid. These secure mainly versus coronary heart problems, as numerous research studies have actually discovered.

Virgin olive oil likewise consists of a lot of anti-oxidants, likewise referred to as phenols. These compounds have a favorable result on the security of the cardiovascular system because they likewise prevent swelling in the body and enhance arterial function.

Because olive oil is a pure source of fat, it likewise consists of no carbs. Because olive oil as unsaturated fatty acid is not as steady as saturated fats at high-temperature levels, the oil is preferably utilized for meals that are prepared on a low flame.

Olive oil is a natural remedy for the prevention of cardiovascular diseases, especially heart attacks and strokes, as well as cancer. The secret is in the record amount of monounsaturated fatty acids Omega-3, which prevent atherosclerotic plaques from being deposited on the walls of blood vessels and even destroy those that already exist.

Accustom yourself to take two tablespoons of olive oil per day (season salad, add to soups, side dishes, marinades), and your heart will work like a clock.

In addition, scientists have found that the oleic acid contained in olive oil stimulates a gene that inhibits the activity of cancer cells. Accordingly, the risk of developing cancer, in particular, breast cancer in women, is reduced.

Butter and cream

Butter and cream contain healthy fatty acids, which is why they should be part of a ketogenic diet. Both contain only a minimal amount of carbohydrates.

Similar to other fatty dairy products, butter and cream also contain a lot of the conjugated linoleic acid, which in turn promotes fat loss. Butter is also one of the most essential ingredients for Bulletproof Coffee - a breakfast drink of the ketogenic diet.

Coconut oil

Coconut oil is an integral part of a ketogenic diet.

Among other things, coconut oil contains medium-chain triglycerides (MCTs). Unlike long-chain fats, MCTs are absorbed directly by the liver and converted to ketones. These in turn act as immediate and fast energy suppliers.

Lauric acid is one of the fatty acids (C 12) that make up the main ingredient in tropical oils such as coconut oil. It is believed that thanks to the mix of MCTs and lauric acid, coconut oil promotes a sustainable state of ketosis. An alternative source of MCTs is concentrated MCT oil.

Berries

Blackberries, strawberries, and raspberries contain fewer carbohydrates than other fruits and contain a lot of useful antioxidants and fiber.

Due to the sugar deprivation in the ketogenic diet, such fruits taste naturally sweet and can be used perfectly as a little snack in between.

Here is an overview of the carbohydrate content for different types of berries (100 grams per serving):

- Blackberries: 10 grams
- Blueberries: 14 grams
- Raspberries: 12 grams
- Strawberries: 8 grams

Unsweetened tea and coffee

Coffee and unsweetened tea contain almost no carbohydrates. For this, they contain caffeine, which has a positive effect on your metabolism and can therefore also directly affect performance, attention, and mood.

Coffee and tea lovers can be happy again: if you consume these drinks regularly in moderation, the risk of developing diabetes is also reduced, according to some studies. The addition of a little whipped cream is also not prohibited. But be careful with reduced-fat versions of finished coffees and teas. These often contain fat-free milk and carbohydrate-rich flavors.

Low-carb yogurt and curd cheese

Greek yogurt or curd is healthy and protein-rich foods. Precisely because they contain a small number of carbohydrates, they can be ideally included in a ketogenic diet. For example, a serving of Greek yogurt (about 150 grams) contains 5 grams of carbohydrates and 11 grams of protein.

Yogurt also regulates appetite and creates a natural feeling of fullness. Ideal for this - a few nuts, cinnamon, and sugar-free sweetener and voila - the perfect ketogenic snack for in between!

Other dairy products

A ketogenic diet often likes to add protein-rich products to a meal. However, try to keep your protein consumption at a moderate level. Most of your meals should include proteins, vegetables, and additional fats or oils.

Raw or organic dairy products should be at the top of the list here. Highly processed foods generally have a carbohydrate content that is 2 to 5 times higher than that of organic milk products.

In addition, it is always better to use full-fat milk products than low-fat variants, since these usually contain more carbohydrates.

Here are a few suggestions as to which dairy products you can incorporate into a ketogenic diet:

Whipped cream

Spreadable fats such as cottage cheese, cream cheese, sour cream, mascarpone, creme fraiche, etc.

Processed cheeses such as mozzarella, brie, blue cheese, Colby or Monterey Jack

Hard cheeses such as cheddar, parmesan, feta, Swiss cheese, etc.

But be careful with the calorie content: Cheese usually already has many calories in small quantities. So, if your focus is on losing weight, then cheese consumption should be reduced somewhat.

HOW TO START YOUR DAY ON KETOGENIC DIET WHEN YOU ARE OVER 50

There is hardly any other meal that is disputed as much as breakfast. Should you have breakfast or not? And if so, which is best? If you eat a ketogenic diet, the question also arises: What can I have breakfast at all? In this book, you will learn everything you need to know about a ketogenic breakfast and ideas of what a ketogenic breakfast can look like.

Ketogenic diet breakfast

"Breakfast is the most important meal of the day." You have probably heard or read this sentence many times. It is based on the idea that after a long period of fasting at night, the body absolutely needs something to eat in the morning in order to get going at all.

Scientifically researched!

The following recipes now give a few examples of what a ketogenic breakfast could look like. There are very simple recipes, some that you can prepare when you don't have much time in the morning, and some that are great for a relaxed ketogenic breakfast.

Ketogenic diet breakfast recipes

Keto Coffee

The middle way in terms of breakfast is keto coffee. Keto coffee contains a lot of fat, hardly any carbohydrates and hardly any protein. This will keep you deep in fat-burning mode, but will also prevent you from starving if you decide to skip breakfast.

(442 kcal; 3g carbohydrates, 2g protein, 49g fat)

Ingredients

- 1 tbsp coconut oil (e.g. Mituso organic coconut oil)
- 1 tbsp butter
- 100 ml coconut milk (e.g. One Nature organic coconut milk)
- 400 ml of hot coffee

Preparation

Mix the ingredients together or mix briefly with a hand blender or blender. Then the coffee becomes particularly creamy.

tip

Experiment with different ingredients until you find your own keto coffee that you like best. You can add different spices, such as cinnamon (e.g. Azafran organic Ceylon cinnamon), cloves (e.g. Sonnentor organic cloves ground) or nutmeg (e.g. eight high organic ground nutmeg).

Instead of coconut milk, you can also use almond milk (e.g. Alpro unsweetened almond milk) or cream. Instead of coconut oil or in addition, you can also use cocoa butter (e.g. Indigo Herbs organic cocoa butter) or MCT oil (e.g. Primal MCT oil).

There are no limits to your imagination, just make sure that your keto coffee contains a lot of fat and little carbohydrates.

You can, of course, use tea instead of coffee. You can also try out different combinations, for example with black tea (e.g. Azafran Indian organic Darjeeling) or chai tea (e.g. Tea Exclusive Masala Chai).

Green keto smoothie

Green smoothies are very nutritious and can also be prepared quickly, can contain very different ingredients and are also ideal for on the go. Ketogenic smoothies are also easy to prepare by avoiding sugary fruit and using berries or avocado instead.

(542 kcal; 5g carbohydrates, 5g protein, 57g fat)

Ingredients

- 3 tbsp coconut oil (e.g. Mituso organic coconut oil)
- 70g avocado
- 30g fresh spinach
- 240ml unsweetened almond milk (e.g. Alpro unsweetened almond milk)
- 100g cucumber

Preparation

Puree all the ingredients in a powerful blender.

If you often make smoothies and want to avoid leftovers, you can prepare the ingredients in large quantities, cut them into small pieces and freeze them in portions. This saves you time and only has to add the liquid.

Eggs with bacon

The classic ketogenic breakfast must not be missing in this recipe collection. Eggs are very healthy, contain many vitamins and taste delicious. They are quickly prepared, highly variable and fill you up for a long time.

(480 kcal; 2g carbohydrates, 29g protein, 39g fat)

Ingredients

- 3 eggs
- 30g bacon in strips
- 1 tbsp coconut oil (e.g. Mituso organic coconut oil)

Preparation

Put the coconut oil in a pan and let it melt. Fry the bacon in the hot pan with the eggs until crispy. You can make scrambled eggs or fried eggs, whichever you prefer.

Keto-muffins

Muffins are easy to prepare and are ideal for on the go. If you like to eat something sweet in the morning, this recipe is for you.

(per serving: 273 kcal; 5g carbohydrates, 8g protein, 24g fat)

Ingredients for 12 servings

- 165g almond flour (e.g. Mea Vita almond flour)
- 65g coarsely ground linseed (e.g. Scharpfenmühle flaxseed)
- 80g erythritol (e.g. Xucker light)
- 2 teaspoons of baking soda
- 1 tsp cinnamon (e.g. Azafran Bio-Ceylon cinnamon)
- ½ tsp salt (e.g. Azafran pink Himalayan salt from Pakistan)
- 30g chopped walnuts (e.g. picked chopped walnuts)
- 6 egg
- 120ml coconut oil (melted but no longer hot) (e.g. Mituso organic coconut oil)
- 120ml coconut milk (e.g. One Nature organic coconut milk)
- 1 lemon

Preparation

Preheat the oven to 170 ° and prepare a muffin tin. Either you use a silicone mold, grease a muffin tin or line it with paper cases.

First mix the dry ingredients, except for the walnuts, in a bowl. Grate the zest of the lemon and mix it with the wet ingredients in another bowl. Then add the dry ingredients and mix everything thoroughly with a mixer or a wooden spoon.

Now fill the muffin tins too full and garnish them with the chopped walnuts. Then bake the muffins for 20-25 minutes, at the end check whether they are baked. To do this, prick a wooden stick in the middle, if it stays clean, they are done. Then let them cool and then remove them from the molds.

Egg Muffins

Egg muffins can be prepared wonderfully. If you don't have much time in the morning, you can pre-cook it 1-2 times a week, keep it in a can in the fridge, and just take it out every morning. Either you eat it cold or you warm it up in the microwave.

(371 kcal per serving; 4g carbohydrates, 23g protein, 19g fat)

Ingredients for 4 servings

- 6 eggs
- 1-2 spring onions (finely chopped)
- 100g cooked ham
- 100g grated cheese
- 1 tsp pesto

Preparation

Chop the ingredients. Mix the eggs with cheese and pesto and spread them in muffin cups, best suited is a muffin tin.

Spread the spring onions and ham evenly over all the muffins. Bake at 180 ° for 20-30 minutes. The egg muffins are also ideal for on the go.

Try other fillings, like spinach with feta, or bacon and cheese, or whatever you can think of.

ketogenic diet breakfast - pancakes

Pancakes are part of an extensive breakfast. With this recipe, you can prepare them ketogenically and you don't have to feel guilty

(515 kcal; 5g carbohydrates, 16g protein, 48g fat)

Ingredients

- 1 tbsp coconut oil (e.g. Mituso organic coconut oil)
- 15g cream cheese
- 2 eggs
- 50g cream
- 30g blueberries

Preparation

Add the oil to the pan and heat. Mix the eggs with the cream cheese and fry in portions in the hot oil. Whip the cream and serve with the blueberries with the pancakes.

For thicker, fluffy pancakes, add 1 tablespoon of coconut flour, ½ teaspoon baking powder and 150 ml almond milk.

Porridge with hemp seeds

You can also prepare this porridge in large quantities. In a closed box, it can be kept in the refrigerator for up to 3 days.

(660 kcal; 15g carbohydrates *, 24g protein, 55g fat)

Ingredients for 2 servings

- 240ml almond milk (e.g. Alpro unsweetened almond milk)
- 75g peeled hemp seeds (e.g. hemp & natural organic hemp seeds peeled)
- 2 teaspoons of chopped linseed (e.g. Scharpfenmühle flaxseed)
- 2 tsp coconut oil (e.g. Mituso organic coconut oil)
- 1 tsp chia seeds (e.g. Naturacereal chia seeds)
- 2-5 drops of Stevia (e.g. Borchert Stevia liquid table sweetness)

- 1 pinch of cinnamon (e.g. Azafran Bio-Ceylon cinnamon)
- 28g ground almonds (e.g. ground Maersch almonds)

Preparation

Put all the ingredients in a saucepan and let them simmer for a few minutes.

You can garnish the porridge with chopped nuts, cinnamon, fresh berries or seeds and enjoy it hot or cold.

* The porridge is relatively high in carbohydrates, but it is almost exclusively fiber that is excreted undigested. Only 3g carbohydrates are processed as sugar per serving.

Ketogenic diet breakfast - sandwich

(483 kcal; 23g protein, 4g carbohydrates, 43g fat)

Ingredients

- 50g cream cheese
- 1 large egg
- 15g ham
- 15g cheese
- 3 slices of cucumber

Preparation

Separate the egg and beat the egg whites until stiff. Mix the egg yolk with the cream cheese and season with a little salt and pepper. Carefully fold the cream cheese and egg yolk mixture under the beaten egg whites.

Place 2 portions on a baking sheet and bake at 150 ° for 20-30 minutes. Brush with the butter and top with the remaining ingredients as desired.

Yogurt with berries

This yogurt is also a quick and easy breakfast that can be easily prepared. It is particularly suitable for those who like some fruit for breakfast.

(214 kcal; 9g carbohydrates, 5g protein, 16g fat)

Ingredients

- 150g Greek yogurt
- 30g berries
- 1 tbsp grated coconut (e.g. Wolfberry organic coconut flakes)

Preparation

Put the yogurt in a bowl, garnish with the berries and the grated coconut. You can use fresh or frozen berries.

To increase the fat content, you can simply drink a cup of coffee with 1-2 tablespoons of coconut oil or add 1-2 tablespoons of MCT oil (e.g. Primal MCT oil) to the yogurt.

Minced meat biscuits

This recipe fits into the "hearty breakfast on the go" category. The cookies are excellent as a snack if you are on the road or traveling longer. They can be kept in the refrigerator, in a closed can, for up to 5 days.

(per biscuit: 47 Kcal, 0.5g carbohydrates, 8g protein, 2g fat)

Ingredients for 18 cookies

- 450g ground beef
- 2 tsp soy sauce (e.g. Kikkoman soy sauce)
- 1 tsp smoked salt (e.g. Krautberger Danish smoked salt)
- 1 tsp ground black pepper (e.g. Wagner spices ground black pepper)
- ½ garlic powder (e.g. Azafran organic garlic granulated)
- ½ tsp paprika powder (e.g. Krautberger gourmet paprika powder noble sweet)

Preparation

Preheat the oven to 170 ° and cover two baking sheets with baking paper. Mix all the ingredients in a bowl, with your hands or a spoon.

Take 1 heaped teaspoon from the mass and shape it into a ball with your hands. Now press the ball flat so that you have around, approx. 5cm large biscuit, which you now place on the baking sheet. Process the remaining minced meat in the same way.

Then put the cookies in the oven, bake them on the middle shelf for 3 hours. Then replace the trays, the top-down and the bottom up, and bake for another 3 hours.

You can also turn the trays during the baking time to ensure that all cookies are baked evenly. In the end, the minced meat biscuits are reminiscent of dried meat. Let them cool for 30 minutes after baking before serving.

You see, there are many different ways in which you can have a ketogenic breakfast. No matter whether you like a hearty or sweet breakfast, on the go or comfortably at the table, fresh every morning or prepare for several days. However, if you want to live an amazing life at

50 then you have to consider any of the above breakfast examples.

Low carb waffles with strawberries

Do you really need a description for this low-carb breakfast? No, just a suitable recipe!

Ingredients:

- 2 eggs, size M
- 2 tablespoons coconut flour
- 2 tablespoons milk
- 1/2 teaspoon baking powder
- 15g xylitol or erythritol

Preparation:

Separate one of the eggs and beat the egg whites until stiff. Fold in the remaining ingredients including the remaining yolk and egg.

Heat the waffle iron and grease well. Bake the waffles for 3 to 4 minutes until they are golden brown. Serve and enjoy with the raspberries.

If you make the waffles the evening before, you can take them to the office or anywhere else. Otherwise, this breakfast idea is, of course, something for the weekend or the day off.

Fried eggs with bacon and onion

Sometimes the simplest things are the best. This is exactly what applies to the fried eggs with bacon and onion.

Simply cut half an onion into half rings and braise in a pan with a few slices of streaky bacon. Then spread everything on the bottom of the pan and beat in two or three eggs.

Fry until the fried eggs meet your own wishes. It goes with raw food, protein bread or roasted vegetables.

Apple with almond butter

Sometimes it has to be quick in the morning. Then this apple with almond butter comes just right.

Simply cut the apple into six to eight pieces, put some almond butter in a small can or bowl and dip and eat the fruit pieces in it.

If you pay close attention to only eating foods that have less than 10 grams of carbohydrates, this low carb breakfast is of course wrong.

However, if you pay attention to the total amount of carbohydrates eaten, you should eat apples regularly. They have a very low-calorie density (little kcal per 100g) and provide micronutrients, fiber, and secondary plant substances.

WEIGHT LOSS AT 50 YEARS AND OLDER

In some cases, you might be on a keto diet plan or even a comparable diet plan such as a low carbohydrate diet plan and still not lose weight. There are a number of factors why you might not lose weight.

Enjoy your protein

Excessive protein is really the most typical error.

A lot of the keto dishes from the net break down the protein requirement for an entire day in simply one meal.

Protein is naturally a fundamental part of your diet plan and you must absolutely cover your protein requires to preserve your muscle mass - specifically if you remain in a calorie deficit.

Too much protein is transformed back into glucose by the body, which is something that you definitely do not desire on a low-carb diet plan!

An excellent standard is 0.8 g protein per kg of your perfect weight on days without a workout.

1g to an optimum of 1.2 g on days with sports.

Numerous physical fitness blog sites typically suggest 2g per kg body weight, which is plainly excessive.

For a short time, just your food digestion suffers - however it can cause kidney and liver issues completely.

Excessive protein is disadvantageous, particularly for ketosis. Do you prevent carbs simply to take in glucose (transformed from excess protein)? Much better not

Consume your fill!

The 2nd most typical error is certainly the extreme calorie deficit!

The very first thing you constantly believe is that you have to consume fewer calories if you desire to lose weight. In addition, less is constantly more when it comes to a diet plan?

NEVER! In order for your body to quit its love handles, you need to offer it sufficient food.

The ideal food, naturally, however certainly enough of it.

Starving him is disadvantageous and causes a scrubby metabolic process and a yo-yo down the spiral.

Shortage informs your body that it needs to bunker. You indicate to it that there is scarcity when you starve your body. Your body wishes to make it through and will save a master in since it does not matter that you wish to reduce weight and there is no threat at all, it just seems that there is insufficient food.

This is likewise the factor why after a diet plan you lose weight once again so rapidly and even put something on leading! You barely consume anything and still do not lose weight - possibly even acquire weight!

You pay so much attention to it - do not consume too much. He has no factor to bring the additional pounds with him!

A calorie deficit must never ever go beyond 10%. If you are not starving on a single day and barely consume anything, this is not an issue.

Consume sufficient veggies, fat, and protein, however not too much and so we come to.

Do not overindulge your appetite!

It holds true that with a properly designed low-carb diet plan you can consume substantially more calories without putting on weight.

That does NOT imply that you can consume an unlimited quantity.

In some books and in lots of groups, the misconception is spread out that you can consume lots of fatty foods with a ketogenic diet plan.

An entire cup of cream is typically put into the coffee and intoxicated with a typical meal. Or consumed an entire pack of mascarpone with berries and nuts for dessert.

A cup of cream has: approx. 620 calories and approx.6.5 g Kh!

A pack of mascarpone has: approx. 800 calories and 8g Kh and here neither berries nor nuts are consisted of!

This is not simply a calorie bomb, however likewise a carbohydrate bomb if you consume keto.

Yes, you need to consume enough, however, this is not a free ticket for unchecked consuming habits!

You do not need to diligently count calories, however, listen to your body!

Consume gradually. Consume yourself complete, however, stop consuming as quickly as you are complete!

Once again, it is not an issue if you eat excessive at your preferred food every once in a while, however, it is bad in the long run.

Eat lots of low-carb vegetables and save on dairy products

I combine these two points because they often go hand in hand. Vegetables are important to you. On the one hand, because it has a strong effect on your satiety, on the other hand, because it is full of important nutrients and vitamins! For the onset of satiety, it is important on the one hand that your stomach is stretched, but on the other hand that you take in enough nutrients.

The first saturation impulses when eating come from the stomach when the stomach wall is stretched by the ingested food. However, filling the stomach alone does not trigger a feeling of satiety. Chemoreceptors register whether enough nutrients are absorbed by the food and report this to the brain. For example, if you fill your stomach with low-calorie liquid, you will not experience a feeling of fullness. If you eat a high-calorie meal, but the volume is very small (such as cheese), the feeling of satiety will also be a long time coming. So the combination of nutrients and sufficient volume is important.

Vegetables have a high volume with a low number of calories and are therefore a wonderful gastric filler.

About half of your plate should be covered with vegetables. If you eat ketogenic or low-carb, make sure you eat low-carb vegetables.

Dairy products have a relatively high amount of carbohydrates.

This will blow up your needs very quickly and there will be no more space for vegetables. Vegetables are not only very important because of the satiating effect, but also because of the vitamins and fiber that they contain.

The protein requirement is also quickly broken up with dairy products. In addition, dairy products trigger cravings in many people and inhibit weight loss. Milk, in general, is "designed" for it to be a small living being, to make it big and strong quickly. To save on dairy products instead of vegetables!

Good fats are important for your body!

With a ketogenic diet, you mostly omit the carbohydrates.

I explained earlier that too much protein is not advisable. And I also talked about fats.

But consuming too few calories is counterproductive when you want to lose weight. That means there is only the fat left that you can screw up to cover your needs adequately. Of course, this does not mean that you can spoon an infinite amount of fat, but another common mistake is often the insufficient amount of fat.

For decades we have been wrongly told that fat is unhealthy and bad. This is also the reason why many people who have understood that good fats are important and healthy are subconsciously still afraid of fat and avoid it.

If you are always hungry, tired and tired, or if you are regularly cold, this is a clear sign that you are too low in fat and you urgently need to increase your amount of fat . Especially in ketosis, fat is your number 1 source of energy and without enough fat, you simply have no energy.

Make sure you eat good fats like virgin coconut oil, MCT oil, pasture-keeping butter, pasture-keeping ghee and extra-virgin olive oil, avocados and avocado oil.

Avoid inferior, high-temperature vegetable fats!

Don't drive yourself crazy!

Stress inhibits weight loss - worse - it promotes weight gain.

Emotional stress too! If you weigh yourself every day, are dissatisfied with yourself and are scared with every bite, then you are driving yourself crazy! This is violent stress for your body that does the opposite of what you want it to do. So banish your scales and don't weigh yourself more than once a week. Listen to your body, pay attention to what you eat and trust that it will work. So you take the stress out of your body and support it in losing weight!

Changing your diet is already stressful for your body, as it does not require additional pressure from you.

Watch out for hidden carbohydrates

Another very common mistake is that you eat products that appear low-carb but are not real. Fitness and low-carb products in particular often advertise with "net carbs" or the "usable carbohydrates" and there is a widespread myth that all polyols / polyhydric alcohols have no usable carbohydrates. But as the title Myth says, the same is not the truth! The only sweetener from the category polyols / polyhydric alcohols that has no usable carbohydrates is erythritol - all others have very usable carbohydrates and effects on blood sugar!

Xylitol, maltitol, isomalt, sorbitol, mannitol, and Co. all have to be counted between 25% and 70%, because unlike erythritol they contain carbohydrates that can be used by the body. In addition to erythritol, xylitol is the only sugar substitute from the polyols category that we recommend in small quantities since it is here that the body absorbs the least amount of carbohydrates.

When buying, make sure that there are no other polyols apart from erythritol and xylitol.

If you pay attention to these sources of error, you should soon be able to lose weight.

If you want to continue supporting your body in losing weight, you can do this as follows:

SUPPLEMENTARY KETO DIET TIPS FOR WOMEN OVER 50

Drink enough water

Especially with a keto diet, it is important to drink a lot. Make sure you drink at least 2 liters a day. If you don't drink enough, your body tends to store water, among other things. Most people often mistake thirst for hunger. Make sure that you are no longer thirsty and you will be less likely to want something to eat.

How much water to drink:

In order to be healthy and feel good during the day, everyone should drink a volume of water that is optimal for their weight. With insufficient water consumption in the body, dehydration can occur, which will be expressed in the form of dry mouth, weakness, headache, high blood pressure, distraction. Therefore, you need to drink enough water, but you need to drink water evenly throughout the day when thirst appears. It is recommended to drink water in its pure form without tea or coffee because they contain dehydrating substances, which lead to the fact that the body removes more moisture than was drunk.

According to the World Health Organization, under normal conditions, to maintain health, an adult should drink at least 30 milliliters of water per kilogram of his body per day. More water should be drunk during physical exertion and playing sports, in hot weather, when drinking alcohol or coffee. Also, for some diseases, for the quick removal of harmful substances from the body, doctors recommend individually drinking more liquid.

The calculation for the amount of water to drink

The minimum amount of water that an adult should drink is calculated by the formula:

The weight of a person in kilograms * 0.03 = the volume of water that a person should drink in liters.

For example, a person weighing 60 kilograms should drink 60 * 0.03 = a minimum of 1.8 liters of water per day to optimally support life and the normal course of all processes in the body during the day.

In children, the body is actively forming, metabolic processes occur faster, so they need to drink more water per kilogram of their weight than adults. Depending on the age of the child, the norm of the volume of water per kilogram of weight changes.

The daily rate of drinking water for a person, depending also on his weight:

Typically, the body itself tells the person when and how much he needs to drink water, causing thirst. But in some cases, a person may not have thirst, but at the same time, his body still needs a daily norm of water. Therefore, it is important to know and ensure that a sufficient amount of water is ingested throughout the day.

Under comfortable conditions, a healthy adult needs to drink at least 30 milliliters of water per kilogram of body weight. The table below shows the daily norms of water, depending on the weight of an adult.

AVERAGE DAILY WATER CONSUMPTION RATES

Adult Weight, kg	Daily rate of water, liters
45	1.35
50	1.5
55	1.65
60	1.8
65	1.95
70	2.1
75	2.25
80	2.4
85	2.55
90	2.7
95	2.85
100	3
105	3.15
110	3.3
115	3.45
120	3.6
125	3.75
130	3.9

135	4.05
140	4.2
145	4.35
150	4.5

The tables above show the average daily water consumption rates. Depending on physical activity, food consumed and environmental conditions, the rate of water consumption may increase. For example, physical activity, alcohol, and hot weather increase the daily intake of water. If a person is thirsty, he must drink water, because thirst - this is the signal of the body that he needs water. Exceptions can be only special types of human illness or being in the postoperative period when the rate of water consumption is regulated by an individual doctor.

Why drink so much water

The body of an adult is 65% water, the human brain contains 75% of the water, 83% in the blood, 76% in the muscles, and 22% in the skeleton. If you drink water less than the daily norm, then dehydration occurs, the proportion of water in the human body drops, the normal functioning of the body is disrupted, metabolic processes slow down, which leads to poor health and illness. A lack of water in the human body can even lead to irreversible aging processes and the appearance of chronic diseases.

Typically, with a lack of water, a person has symptoms such as pain in various organs, heartburn, indigestion, nausea and vomiting, bad breath, talking in a dream, fatigue, irritability, anxiety, heaviness in the head and a rush of blood to the face.

The lack of water in the human body leads to a decrease in metabolic processes, which leads to the accumulation of fats, slowing down the regeneration and reproduction of new cells in the body. The release of toxins and harmful substances from the body is slowed down, the human body is slagged, from which various diseases appear. Nails and hair become brittle, the skin dries and ages. The digestive system suffers, which is manifested in the appearance of constipation, heaviness in the abdomen, discomfort in the intestines. The body experiences stress, which affects the nervous and system and mental state of a person.

Do not bring the body to a state of dehydration. If the body is thirsty, then you need to drink water. Care should be taken to ensure that water is always at hand to quench your thirst. It is necessary to control the daily water intake so that it is within the normal range. This will ensure the normal functioning of the body, health and good mood.

It is especially important to drink plenty of fluids for those who want to lose weight. Often the cause of excess weight is a violation of the water-salt balance and slagging of the body. Drinking the daily norm of water will help restore the water-salt balance, remove toxins from the body and normalize metabolic processes. But you should not drink excessively much liquid, you just need to consume the daily rate of water per kilogram of weight, as indicated in the table above. Drinking water within the recommended range will contribute to weight loss.

How to drink water:

In order to enhance the benefits of water for the body, it is recommended to adhere to simple rules when using it:

- Drink a glass of water on an empty stomach.
- Drink water evenly throughout the day.
- Drink water 15 minutes before eating.
- Drink water at room temperature.
- Drink only clean, filtered and boiled water.
- Follow the daily recommended water intake per kilogram of weight.
- Drink water with honey or lemon.

Water and lemon

To enhance the beneficial qualities of water, freshly squeezed lemon juice or honey can be diluted in it. These two ingredients are a storehouse of vitamins and minerals that have a beneficial effect on the body.

Lemon in large quantities contains not only vitamin C, which stimulates the immune system but also many other vitamins and nutrients. Water with lemon is useful in that it improves immunity, saturates the body with a large number of vitamins, macro- and microelements.

Honey is a storehouse of useful substances important for the normal functioning of the body. It is recommended to dilute a teaspoon of honey in a glass of clean water. Water with honey is useful in that it nourishes the body with a large number of useful substances, encourages, gives strength.

It is recommended to drink water with lemon or honey on an empty stomach in order to cleanse the gastrointestinal system from toxins and toxins, saturate the body with useful substances and rather wake up. Also, drinking water with lemon or honey contributes to weight loss.

Water with lemon or honey is good for all people with some exceptions. Water with lemon is contraindicated in people with gastric ulcers, as it can cause ulcer irritation. Water with honey is contraindicated for allergy sufferers since honey contained in water can cause an allergic reaction.

Eat spicy

Chilli also helps to stimulate your metabolism. Hot spices can also help lower insulin levels. A high insulin level favors fat storage. The mild spiciness of ginger can also help because it also stimulates digestion and helps drain the body.

Move more

Don't worry, you don't have to start a marathon because a little more activity in your life can do a lot. Prefer the stairs instead of the elevator. Walk short distances on foot or by bike or take a relaxing walk if you would normally watch TV. Not only will your weight benefit - but you will also feel more energetic.

Get enough salt!

With a low-carb and ketogenic diet, your body excretes a lot more salt. But salt is an important electrolyte that your body needs. Too little salt also leads to water retention. In addition, it also leads to worse side effects such as headache, fatigue, dizziness and constipation. Provide your body with sufficient salt, at least 2-4g per day.

Sleep enough

Sleeping too little is a stress factor for your body and, as you already know, stress is rather unfavorable for weight loss. In addition, a night of sufficient and restful sleep is important for a balanced hormone balance, which plays an important role in regulating your weight.

Why is sleep so important?

About a third of our lives we spend on sleep. To understand why sleep is important, think of your body like a factory that performs a number of vital functions. When you fall asleep, your body begins a "night shift":

- Restoration of damaged cells that were exposed to ultraviolet rays, stress, etc.
- Restoration of muscle tissue injuries;
- Increase immunity;

- Recovery after daily activity;
- Preparation of the heart and cardiovascular system for the next day.

When you do not get enough sleep, you gradually become more vulnerable. Lack of sleep harms the body - both in the short and long term. The wakefulness mode gets lost, the concentration of attention decreases, memory worsens. You feel tired, productivity drops, depression gradually develops. Scientists from Waseda University of Japan and Kao Corporation believe that overweight, obesity, and diabetes are the consequences of regular sleep deprivation. Earlier this phenomenon was noted by Swedish scientists.

Deep sleep concept

There are two main phases of sleep:

slow sleep (nap, light sleep, deep sleep);

REM sleep (activation of all processes in the body before waking up).

Deep sleep is most important because it is during this phase that the body recovers and accumulates energy.

Deep sleep is the phase of sleep in which the heartbeat and breathing slow down. Your body relaxes completely, and you hardly move. This is the most important sleep cycle. If you find yourself waking sluggishly, even if you spent seven or eight hours in bed, your sleep may not have been deep enough.

The duration of the deep sleep phase changes throughout life. Babies and toddlers need to sleep much more than older children. By the age of five, most children have typical adult sleep patterns.

How much does an adult need to sleep to get enough sleep?

A clear answer, what is the norm of sleep for an adult, is impossible. All people are different, and the need for sleep in each watch depends on many factors: age, body characteristics, frequency of physical activity, lifestyle, etc.

Six hours of sleep is enough for someone to feel sleepy and awake. And for someone, vivacity comes only after 10 hours of sleep.

You probably heard the phrase "geniuses sleep little." Usually, it is supported by facts from history. For example, it is believed that the Roman politician and commander Guy Julius Caesar allocated only three hours a day for sleep. The artist and inventor Leonardo da Vinci slept 15-20 minutes every four hours, which means that it took 2 hours to sleep just a day

But about the legendary physicist Albert Einstein they say that he could sleep for 10-12 hours, believing that a full deep sleep is a key to a clear mind and genius.

So still, how much does an adult need to sleep per day? Below are the average values of the required amount of sleep for each age. Scientists of the National Sleep Fund during a two-year study have deduced the average value of sleep needs in hours at different ages.

How much sleep does a woman over 50 need

It is believed that women should sleep an odd number of hours, and men even. For women, the duration of sleep is important. They need to sleep a little more than men, at least 20 minutes. This fact is explained by the ability of women to simultaneously focus on several tasks at once.

Healthy Sleep Rules

We have already figured out how many hours a normal sleep for a person should last approximately. But so that it really benefits and becomes for you a source of well-being and vitality for the whole day, you should organize your principles or rituals of healthy sleep.

There are several common principles for quality sleep:

- Get up and go to bed every day at the same time;
- Do not lie in bed after waking up - it is better to try to get up the first time and start your day;
- At least an hour before bedtime, organize a calm atmosphere around you without fuss, loud sounds, and bright light;

- Do not fall asleep under the tv. If you already have such a habit, then try to unlearn. Try not to fall asleep to the sound and glow of the tv, turn on pleasantly pleasant music in the style of light jazz or "relaxation";
- Do not eat at least 2-3 hours before bedtime;
- Physical activities during the day contribute to quality sleep;
- Before going to bed, give up alcohol, coffee, and cigarettes;
- Before going to bed, ventilate the room. Fresh air will help you fall asleep more quickly.

What time should I go to bed?

The physiological and biochemical processes of the body are subject to circadian rhythms. Simply put, with the advent of dawn, our brain wakes up, the work of all sensory organs begins and is maintained until sunset. This is the concept of circadian rhythms. Therefore, it is better to go to bed before midnight, since from 12 a.m. to 5 a.m., our body temperature decreases, activity drops, the body needs rest. Even if you work at night, your biological clock operates as usual.

Is it good to sleep during the day?

Everyone who went to kindergarten remembers how he wanted to jump, run, play - do anything, but just not sleep after dinner. However, the teachers categorically insisted and sent all the children in bed. Now, taking a nap in the afternoon is the dream of many adults.

Let's look at how daytime sleep affects the body. It may turn out that formidable educators from our memories were right.

Specialists in the study of the benefits of sleep have shown that afternoon siesta has a positive effect on our body in psychological and physical aspects. NASA pilots acted as experimental. The results of the study showed that a 26-minute pilot siesta improves performance by 34% and attentiveness by 54%.

Daytime Duration:

From 2 to 5 minutes - micro-nap. Effectively combats drowsiness;

From 5 to 20 minutes - a mini-nap. Increases alertness, endurance, performance;

20 minutes is a really good dream. It has the advantages of micro- and mini-naps, improves muscle memory and "cleanses" the brain of unnecessary information;

It is believed that midday sleep for 20 minutes is optimal and beneficial for a healthy person, as it serves as a good prevention of physical and mental fatigue.

A siesta lasting more than 40 minutes is more likely to do harm than to help overcome drowsiness. A team of doctors from the American College of Cardiology found that if you sleep for more than 40 minutes during the day, a metabolic disorder (metabolic syndrome) can occur.

For people with insomnia and severe depression, it is best to give up daytime sleep: in this state, it will be more difficult to control yourself and you can sleep for several hours.

7 DAYS KETO MEAL PLAN 1

The following diet plan is an exemplary 7-day ketogenic meal plan. This weekly schedule can be adjusted according to your individual preferences as long as you do not consume more than 30-50g carbohydrates per day.

Monday

Breakfast: two eggs fried in butter with a green salad.

Noon: Minced meatballs with cheese, mushrooms, and avocado on a salad.

In the evening: pork chops fried with green beans in coconut oil.

Tuesday

Breakfast: omelet with mushrooms.

Noon: Tuna salad with celery and tomatoes on a green salad.

In the evening: Fried chicken breast strips with cream sauce and broccoli.

Wednesday

Breakfast: stuffed peppers with cheese and eggs.

Noon: rocket salad with hard-boiled eggs, turkey, avocado and blue cheese.

In the evening: grilled salmon fillet sautéed with spinach in coconut oil.

Thursday

Breakfast: Greek yogurt with flax seeds and blueberries.

Lunch: steaks with cauliflower rice, cheese, herbs, avocado, and salsa dip.

In the evening: shrimp with zucchini cubes and spinach fried in coconut oil.

Friday

Breakfast: baked avocado on a bed of lettuce.

Noon: Caesar salad with strips of chicken breast.

In the evening: pork chops with vegetables.

Saturday

Breakfast: Baked cauliflower toast with cheese and avocado.

Noon: salmon fillet with spinach and green salad.

In the evening: minced meatballs served with zucchini noodles and parmesan.

Sunday

Breakfast: coconut milk chia pudding with coconut flakes and walnuts.

Noon: salad plate made from vegetables, hard-boiled eggs, avocado, cheese, and turkey.

In the evening: chicken curry with coconut milk.

7 DAYS KETO MEAL PLAN 2

Monday

Breakfast: 2 boiled eggs, 30 gr cheese, protein shake 50 gr., coffee

Noon: 30 gr almonds, Apple

In the evening: 170 grams of stewed chicken breast, 150 gr. lettuce

Tuesday

Breakfast: 3 egg omelet, beetroot salad 150 gr., Coffee

Noon: Smoothie with nuts, milk and cottage cheese (30 g. Nuts, 200 ml. Milk, 50 g. Cottage cheese)

In the evening: 200 gr. roast beef, stewed zucchini 150 gr.

Wednesday

Breakfast: 1 egg, half an avocado, 150 gr. baked salmon with vegetables

Noon: Cheese balls with yogurt (150 ml of yogurt, 30 g. Balls)

In the evening: 200 gr. baked turkey with cheese and herbs.

Thursday

Breakfast: Two egg omelet with fried bacon and cheese, coffee

Lunch: Protein shake 40 gr., grapefruit

In the evening: 200 gr. baked meat, salad 150 gr.

Friday

Breakfast: Fried eggs from two eggs with mushrooms and cheese, coffee

Noon: Vegetable sticks (3-5 pcs.)

In the evening: Pork steak 200 gr., stewed vegetables 100 gr.

Saturday

Breakfast: Three egg omelet with cheese, green salad, coffee

Noon: 30 gr pistachios

In the evening: 170 gr beef stew, boiled broccoli 150 gr.

Sunday

Breakfast: Smoked salmon with baked tomatoes 250 gr., 1 boiled egg

Noon: Smoothie with milk, nuts and cottage cheese (50 g. Cottage cheese, 30 g. Nuts, 200 ml. Milk)

In the evening: 150 gr. fried pork with vegetables

KETO 30 DAYS MEAL PLAN

	Breakfast	Dinner	Dinner
Day 1	Eggs with spinach and crepes	Chicken and Almond Sandwich	Eggplant Lasagna
Day 2	Low carb pancakes	Avocado, Egg and Tuna Salad	Spinach and Bacon Chicken
Day 3	Hotcakes	Bacon Shrimp	Shrimps in a creamy garlic sauce
Day 4	Beef Empanadas	Cheeseburger with Bacon and Mushrooms	Stuffed chicken breasts
Day 5	Spinach Omelet	Salad rolls with ground beef	Chicken schnitzel
Day 6	Egg and Vegetable Frittata	Stuffed jalapenos	Sausages with String Beans

Day 7	Ham and Cheese Hot Cakes	Asparagus in bacon	Eggplant Salad
Day 8	Almond Flour Keto Donuts	Zucchini bread with cheese	Filet Mignon with Bacon
Day 9	Cauliflower Cheese Bread	Lamb and bacon cutlets	Chicken with Lemon Sauce
Day 10	Keto Buns	Fried chicken slices	Meatloaf with bacon
Day 11	Pancakes with yogurt and berries	Bacon Meatballs	Alfredo with Chicken and Broccoli
Day 12	Broccoli Cheese Bread	Salmon Sushi Rolls	Buffalo Chicken Wings
Day 13	Coconut Milk Avocado Smoothie	Spinach Chicken	Nachos with ground beef and guacamole

Day 14	Coconut Pancakes	Keto Pizza	Chicken Cordon Bleu
Day 15	Ground Beef Omelet	Focaccia with garlic and herbs	Cabbage Dumplings with Ginger and Pork
Day 16	Fried eggs with leek	Stuffed avocado	Spinach Shrimps in Alfredo Sauce
Day 17	Light Keto Pancakes	Mushrooms with Bacon and Cheese	KFC style fried chicken
Day 18	Almond Flour Keto Donuts	Zucchini pasta with chicken	Mexican tacos with cheese
Day 19	Syrniki	Egg salad with tahini and mayonnaise.	Jalapeno Chicken Casserole
Day 20	Eggs with asparagus	Stuffed cabbage	Shrimp Zucchini Pasta

Day 21	Cupcakes with avocado, egg, and cheese.	Chicken and Almond Sandwich	Stuffed Lasagna Peppers
Day 22	Baked Avocado with Egg	Chicken with Pesto and Mozzarella	Baked Shrimp with Asparagus
Day 23	Portobello Stuffed Mushrooms	Cheese balls	Eggplant Lasagna
Day 24	Cheese omelet with bacon and mushrooms	Zucchini tacos with beef and cheese	Grilled Beef Steak Ribeye
Day 25	Boiled eggs with spices	Shrimp Broccoli	Low Carb Pizza
Day 26	Almond and Coconut Bread	Portobello Stuffed Mushrooms	Brisket with eggplant, zucchini, and spinach

Day 27	Omelet with mushrooms and cottage cheese	Tortilla with beef and avocado	Stuffed Zucchini with Bacon
Day 28	Low-Carbon Vegetable Pie	Coconut Canapé Pizza	Zucchini noodles with meatballs
Day 29	Zucchini Cupcakes	Fritatta with spinach and mushrooms	Beef and Eggplant Kebab
Day 30	Cauliflower pancakes	Greek Keto Salad	Chicken Cordon Bleu